AN ANALYTICAL STUDY OF PULMONARY FUNCTIONS IN HEALTHY YOUNG ADULTS OF DIFFERENT MIZAJ

By

DANISH KAMAAL CHISHTI

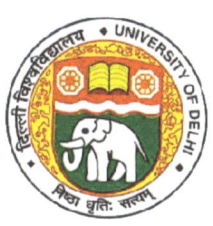

Dissertation submitted to the
University of Delhi

In partial fulfillment
of the requirements for the degree of

MAHIR-E- TIB
(DOCTOR OF MEDICINE)

In

MUNAFE-UL- AZA
(PHYSIOLOGY)

Supervisor
Prof. Yusuf Jamal

Co Supervisor
Dr Shabbir Ahmad

Book Details

Paperback: 94 pages
Publisher: IS Independent Publishing Platform; 1st edition (January, 2015)
Language: English
ISBN-10: 150598758X
ISBN-13: 978-1505987584
Product Dimensions: 6 x 9 inches

Printed IS Publishing
eStore address
An Amazon.com Company
IS Independent Publishing Platform
Made in USA

University of Delhi, New Delhi

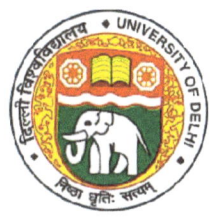

<u>DECLARATION BY THE CANDIDATE</u>

I hereby declare that the dissertation entitled **"An Analytical Study of Pulmonary Functions in Healthy Young Adults of Different Mizaj"** is an original and genuine research work carried out by me under the guidance of **Prof. Yusuf Jamal,** HOD, **Department of Munafe-ul-Aza, A & U Tibbia College Karol Bagh, New Delhi as Supervisor** and **Dr Shabbir Ahmad** as co supervisor.

DANISH KAMAAL CHISHTI)

Ayurvedic and Unani Tibbia College
Karol Bagh, New Delhi 110005

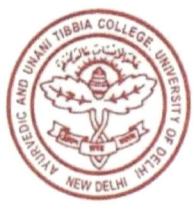

CERTIFICATE

This is to certify that the dissertation entitled **"An Analytical Study of Pulmonary Functions in Healthy Young Adults of Different Mizaj"** is a bonafide research work done by **Danish Kamaal Chishti** in partial fulfillment of the requirement for the degree of **Mahir-e-Tib** (**Doctor of Medicine**) in **Munafe-ul-Aza** under our direct supervision and guidance.

All the observations reported in this dissertation have been checked and verified by us from time to time. This dissertation contains ample evidences of original thoughts and specific data. Therefore this dissertation is being submitted to the adjucators for adjudication.

Supervisor: **Co-supervisor**
Prof. Dr Yusuf Jamal   **Dr Shabbir Ahmed**

Department of Munafe-ul-Aza (Physiology)
A & U Tibbia College
Karol Bagh

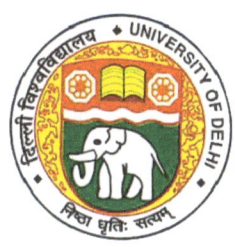

COPYRIGHT

Declaration by the Candidate

I hereby declare that the University of Delhi, New Delhi shall have the rights to preserve, use and disseminate this dissertation in print or electronic format for academic / research purpose.

(DANISH KAMAAL CHISHTI)

Abstract

Mizaj is one of the foremost and basic concepts of *Unani* medicine. Diagnosis and line of treatment of a disease are based on *Mizaj* of the patient and the drugs given for the treatment. Every human being has been endowed a specific *Mizaj* upon which structures and functions of his body are dependent. If the *Mizaj* of a person is changed his functions as well as structures tend to change. There are some factors responsible for alteration of the *Mizaj* like age, diet, weather, residence, occupation and habit. These factors play an important role in changing the *Mizaj* and in causing diseases in an individual. For example, the persons of *Barid Mizaj* (cold temperament) are generally susceptible to develop *Suddah* (obstruction) in the body and obesity etc. Similarly the persons of *Har Mizaj* (hot temperament) will be prone to hot diseases like fever etc. Therefore, for maintaining health it is necessary to find out the *Mizaj* of the patient, disease and the drugs given for the treatment. By the assessment of *Mizaj* of an individual and the changing factors we can predict about health status and the diseases for which individual is more prone to develop in future.

Objective of the study was to find out the range of pulmonary functions in Healthy Young Adults of Different Mizaj.

The present study is cross sectional. Total 100 healthy young adults fulfilling the criteria were enrolled in the study. Following enrolment of the volunteers, their *Mizaj* were assessed by two predetermined proforma that were based on objective and subjective parameters given by Eminent Unani physicians i.e. *A'lamat Ajnase A'shra* (ten determinants) and *A'lamat Ghalbae Akhlat* (signs and symptoms of dominance of Humour).

In the present study, our emphasis was on *Mizaj* of individual and *its relation with pulmonary functions*, therefore, the present concordance between *Mizaj* and pulmonary functions in young healthy adults was evaluated. Further study on large scale is needed to determine relationship between *Mizaj* and pulmonary functions considering the factors responsible for change in the Mizaj.

Key words: *Mizaj*; Unani System of Medicine.

CONTENTS

INTRODUCTION

Everybody wants to maintain health, but nobody knows about the factors which provide for that. It is nothing but it is the *Mizaj* of an individual. The word *'Mizaj'*, used in the Unani system of medicine, is so papular that not only the Unani physicians are aware about it but also general people, either they are literate or illiterate, are well familiar with its name and meaning. *Mizaj* is the quality or power produced in the compound after intermixing of *Ustaqissat e Arba'* (four elements) with their equal or unequal quantities which is equally distributed in the whole compound. This is the quality which provides a power to the compound, because of which the compound performs its functions. If this quality or power of the compound is good, normal functions will be produced from it and vice versa. The *Mizaj* or power of the compound depends upon the quantities and qualities of *Ustaqissat e Arba'* that participate in the formation of the compound. When these elements intermix with each other, in the compound, with suitable or appropriate quantities and qualities as per need of the compound, as a result a specific *Mizaj* is formed in the same which is suitable for its normal functioning and the other round. There are nine types of *Mizaj*, one is *Mo'tadil* (normal or balanced) and eight are *Ghair Mo'tadil* (*Tibbi Mo'tadil*) (abnormal or imbalanced) four *Mufrad* (simple) and four *Murakkab* (compound). For example, if the dominant element (part) in the compound is *Nar* (fire), the compound would be considered as of *Har Mizaj* (hot temperament). Similarly, if the dominant element or part of the compound is *Maa* (water), the compound would be considered as of *Barid Mizaj* (clod temperament). Likewise *Ratab* and *Yabis Mizaj* are obtained from dominance of *Hawa* (air) and *Arz* (soil) respectively.

Similarly, if two elements out of four *Ustaqissat* (fire, air, water and soil) become dominant, the compound would be

9

called by their qualities. For example, if fire and air both are dominant together in the compound, it would be considered as *Har Ratab*. Like wise, there are four types of *Murakkab Mizaj* as *Har Ratab, Har Yabis, Barid Ratab* and *Barid Yabis*. Because of intermixing of elements in different proportion in the different compounds, numbers of *Mizaj* may exceed the 9 and can reach beyond the limit of counting. That's why each individual has its specific *Mizaj*.

Human being is also considered as a *Murakkab* (compound) and gets its *Mizaj* (temperament) in uterus in the form of *Nutfa* (zygote) after intermixing of *Madda e Manviyah* with each other. These *Madda e Manviyah* are also made from *Ustaqissat e Arba'* i.e. *Juze Nari, Juze Hawaee, Juze Maee* and *Juze Arzi*. If these *Ajza e Manviyah* are intermixed with proper quantities and qualities, an appropriate compound (foetus) is formed having *Mizaj e Asli* as *Mizaj e Mo'tadil,* As a result the structures of growing foetus will be proportionate anatomically and functions will be normal and the foetus or a child will carry a good health and good character, and when these *Ajza e Manviyah* do not intermix with each other in proper quantity, as a result *Mizaj e Asli* will not be *Mo'tadil* and the *Sakht* (structure) and the *Afa'al* of the body will be abnormal, because of which so many kinds of congenital deformities may be developed in baby in place of health i.e., if the *Madda e Manviyah* (semen) is less or more in quantity, foetus will not be developed properly. If *Madda e Manviyah* is less in quantity, any organ may be smaller in size such as "Microcephaly". Similarly, if the quantity of *Maadda e Manviah* is more, The related organ of the body may became enlarged such as "Macrocephaly" . There are so many kinds of congenital diseases that develop in foetus due to change in the genetic material (chromosomes and genes) like, Down's syndrome, Klinefelter's syndrome, Turner's syndrome, PKU (phenylketonurea), Tay-sachs disease, galactosemia etc. Till now, over 2300 hereditary diseases have been identified. If a person is born with such *Mizaj e Asli* that has deviated towards *Sue Mizaj* but is not out of the range of *Mizaj e Mo'tadil Shakhsi*, he will be more prone to develop such diseases having same *Mizaj* as of foetus. That's why, a close relationship between temperament and disease of the patient is observed. People of one type of temperament may be prone to develop a particular group of diseases in different stages of life and under different climatic conditions. For example, a person of cold temperament is generally prone to obesity and of hot temperament is prone to acute fever, heat stroke, dehydration, hypertension etc. There are some factors, having their specific temperament, responsible for influencing the temperament of an individual and causing diseases like age, air, place (residence of an individual), season, diet and occupation. If persons having *Mizaj Har* adopt *Har Tadabeer,* they may develop diseases like *Humma e Yaum,* acute fever, heat stroke, dehydration, hypertension, diabetes, increased thirst, insomnia, weak digestion, soft and delicate constitution of body. Similarly, if a person having *Mizaj Barid* and gets *Barid Tadabeer,* he will be more susceptible to develop diseases like *Humma e Balghamiah,* decreased metabolism, obesity, *Suddah* (obstruction) which may cause so many diseases in the body for example, if *Suddah* (obstruction) occurs in the brain vessels, it may causes *Falij* (paralysis). If it occurs in the vessels of the heart, it may cause angina and MI (myocardial infarction). If obstruction occurs in the arteries supplying genital organs infertility may be developed. If *Suddah* occurs in deep vein of the body, it may cause deep vein thrombosis. *Sue Mizaj Barid* is the most common cause of *Aa'sabi Amraz* (Nervine diseases) like *Isterkha, Ra`sha, Ikhtilaj, Khadar, Falij, Laqwah* etc. There are some other diseases which may develop because of *Sue Mizaj Barid* as cough and common cold, *Buhtus Saut* (hoarseness of voice), Asthma, Ascites etc. The persons having *Mizaj Ratab* if adopt *Ratab Tadabeer*, they may acquire some diseases as *Hummae Balghamiah*, infections (frequently), laziness, *Buhtus Saut* (hoarseness of voice), increased sleep, heart pain, *Zo'fe Hazm* (dyspepsia), general weakness, prolonged fever, diarrhoea, piles, dysmenorrhoea, ulcers, fistulae, epilepsy, stomatitis. Similarly, the persons having *Sue Mizaj Yabis* when adopt *Yabis Tadabeer* they may be susceptible to produce diseases of *Sue Mizaj Yabis* i.e. *Humma e Ruba'*, *Laghri* (leanness)[3], asthma, anosmia, body ache, *Zo'fe Aa'za* and male infertility.

Everything (animate or inanimate), which is present in this world has its own specific *Mizaj*. Like this, each and every individual has specific kinds of *Mizaj* but these are suitable for them. Not only the human being having its specific temperament but also a species, race and organs of the body are furnished distinct temperament that are *Mo'tadil* (suitable) for them. For example, Africans and Indians having their specific *Mizaj* which differs from each other, but are suitable for their body functions i.e. if African temperament is replaced by Indian temperament, it will be harmful for them and they will feel discomfort and cannot adjust themselves with that. Same like this, if an organ having *Mizaj e Asli* as *Mizaj e Har* acquired *Mizaj e Barid,* it will lose its harmony; as a result abnormal functions will be manifested from it. There are some factors responsible for change in temperaments of human being like age, place or residence, weather, diets, *tadabeer* (regimens), occupation and habit etc. Out of all these factors, everyone has its specific *Mizaj*. Therefore, for maintaining health of an individual and avoidance of disease, it is necessary to be acquainted with these factors and their temperament. Following assessment of *Mizaj* of human being and the factors responsible for changing the *Mizaj,* we can predict about the health status of an individual as well as of a community in a region or a country for example a person having *Mizaje Barid* and adopts cold *Tadabeer* like cold diet, stays in cold place and cold weather, surely he will fall ill. And when he reaches *Sinne Kuhoolat* and *Sinne Shaikhookhat,* he will not pass his life as better as that of the persons having *Sue Mizaj Har,* and he would fall ill frequently and vice versa. Similarly, if a person having *Sue Mizaj Ratab* and use *Ratab Tadabeer,* he will frequently feel discomfort in comparison of the person having *Sue Mizaj Yabis.*

In this way, we may get to know about the health status of a community and an epidemiology of diseases in a region or a country as a whole, following determination of *Mizaj* of the region, because every region or country influences the *Mizaj* of its inhabitants, due to which they become susceptible to develop some specific diseases i.e. inhabitants of *Masakine Harrah* (hot places) usually suffer from digestive problems and more loss of *Rutoobate Badan* (body fluids) because of which they shortly become cold. Similarly, inhabitants of *Masakine Rataba* (wet places) usually tend to be obese and more susceptible to develop chronic fever, *Ishal* (diarrhoea), piles, menorrhagia, infections and epilepsy etc. As far as seasons are concerned, each season has its specific *Mizaj* and causes some specific diseases in the persons having same *Mizaj* as that of the season. For example, in winter season, persons with *Balghami Mizaj* develop more *Balghami Amraz* like, *Zukam* (common cold), pleurisy, *Buhtus Saut,* backache, neurological diseases etc. than that of the persons having *Mizaj e Har.*

Unani medicine is distinct in its concept of disease and health. Both disease and health are described in the context of *Mizaj* and *Sakht* (structure) harmony, when both *Mizaj* and *Sakht* are in harmony with the environmental demands then the state is called health. *Mizaj* imparts a shape, the most suitable for performing the *Mizaji* functions in a given environment. *Sakht* and its inherent capacities mediate the concordance between the *Mizaji* functions and environmental demand to establish a state

13

of optimum adjustment and survival. Regarding disease causation, Unani physicians recognised a relationship between *Mizaj, Sakht* and environment, and thus relieved the medicine from the sling of demon dominance, demon entry, and influence of evil spirit and influence of evil eyes.

In Unani System of Medicine diagnosis and treatment are based on *Mizaj* of the patients and the drugs are given to the patient. Therefore, for maintaining health and treatment of disease it is mandatory to determine the *Mizaj* of patients and disease. Like finger prints which are used to identify a person, similarly by determination of *Mizaj*, we can find out *Halate Badan* (health and disease condition of the body). If we are aware about the temperament of an individual and the factors mentioned above, we can maintain the health and can treat the disease, by giving some instructions/ knowledge and drugs as per their temperaments. By doing this, we can improve health status and life expectancy of human beings at individual, community and country levels. Keeping these points in mind present study was carried out with one year duration.

Objective of the present study were to assess the *Mizaj* of the young healthy adults having different types of *Mizaj* and to evaluate the ratio of pulmonary functions in respect of *Mizaj* and then to provide some knowledge/instructions to maintain their health and to prevent the diseases which may occur in future. For the assessment of *Mizaj* two proforma were used, designed by eminent Unani physicians. One was based on *Alamat Ajnase Ashra* and other was based on signs and symptoms of dominance of *Akhlat* (body fluids).

By *Alamate Ajnase A'shra, Mizaj e Khilqi* is determined whereas *Khilti* dominance reflects the present status of the body. Depending on the *Tadabeer* adopted *Khilti Mizaj* may or may not be commensurating with *Mizaj e Asli* or *Khilqi*.

14

OBJECTIVES

1. To assess the *Mizaj* of the young healthy adults.
2. To evaluate the relationship of pulmonary functions in respect of *Mizaj* of the adults.
3. To provide some knowledge/instructions for prevention of other diseases related to the *Mizaj* of the adults.

LITERATURE REVIEW

Pulmonary function tests

Pulmonary function tests (PFTs) are noninvasive diagnostic tests that provide measurable feedback about the function of the lungs by assessing lung volumes, capacities, rates of flow and gas exchange. A normally-functioning pulmonary system operates on many different levels to ensure adequate balance. One of the primary functions of the pulmonary system is ventilation, the movement of air into and out of the lungs. Some medical conditions may interfere with ventilation. These conditions may lead to chronic lung disease. Conditions that interfere with normal ventilation are categorized as restrictive or obstructive. An obstructive condition occurs when air has difficulty flowing out of the lungs due to resistance, causing a decreased flow of air. A restrictive condition occurs when the chest muscles are unable to expand adequately, creating a disruption in air flow. Pulmonary function tests may be indicated to determine the presence, location, cause, and characteristics of the problem, and to guide treatment.[1]

Pulmonary function tests are an inclusive term that refers to several different procedures that measure lung function in different ways. Some of the more common values that may be measured during pulmonary function testing include:

- Tidal volume (TV): This is the amount of air inhaled or exhaled during normal breathing.

- Minute volume (MV): This is the total amount of air exhaled per minute.

- Vital capacity (VC): This is the total volume of air that can be exhaled after maximum inspiration.

- Functional residual capacity (FRC): This is the amount of air remaining in lungs after normal expiration.

- Total lung capacity (TLC): This is the total volume of lungs when maximally inflated.

- Forced vital capacity (FVC): This is the amount of air exhaled forcefully and quickly after maximum inspiration.

- Forced expiratory volume (FEV): This is the volume of air expired during the first, second, and third seconds of the FVC test.

- Forced expiratory flow (FEF). This is the average rate of flow during the middle half of the FVC test.

- Peak expiratory flow rate (PEFR). This is the maximum volume during forced expiration.

Spirometry:

Spirometry is a physiological test that measures how an individual inhales or exhales volumes of air as a function of time. The primary signal measured in Spirometry may be volume or flow. Spirometry is invaluable as a screening test of general respiratory health in the same way that blood pressure provides important information about general cardiovascular health. However, on its own, Spirometry does not lead clinicians directly to an etiological diagnosis. Some indications for Spirometry are given in table 1. In this document, the most important aspects of Spirometry are the forced vital capacity (FVC), which is the volume delivered during expiration made as forcefully and completely as possible starting from full inspiration, and the forced expiratory volume (FEV) in one second, which is the volume delivered in the first second of an

FVC maneuvers. Other Spirometric variables derived from the FVC maneuvers are also addressed. Spirometry can be undertaken with many different types of equipment, and requires cooperation between the subject and the examiner, and the results obtained will depend on technical as well as personal factors. If the variability of the results can be diminished and the measurement accuracy can be improved, the range of normal values for populations can be narrowed and abnormalities more easily detected. The Snowbird workshop held in 1979 resulted in the first American Thoracic Society (ATS) statement on the standardization of spirometry.[2]

Indications for spirometry
Diagnostic
To evaluate symptoms, signs or abnormal laboratory tests
To measure the effect of disease on pulmonary function
To screen individuals at risk of having pulmonary disease
To assess pre-operative risk
To assess prognosis
To assess health status before beginning strenuous physical activity
Programmes
Monitoring
To assess therapeutic intervention
To describe the course of diseases that affect lung function
To monitor people exposed to injurious agents
To monitor for adverse reactions to drugs with known pulmonary toxicity
Disability/impairment evaluations
To assess patients as part of a rehabilitation programme
To assess risks as part of an insurance evaluation
To assess individuals for legal reasons
Public health
Epidemiological surveys
Derivation of reference equations
Clinical research

Table 1: Indications for Spirometry

A spirometer can be used to measure movement of air in and out of the lungs. Analysis of data on volume and flow can be used by doctors to distinguish different types of respiratory conditions. Measurements can be compared to expected values. Spirometers differ in the methods used to obtain breathing measurements and in the range of measurements that they can take. They also vary considerably in reliability, accuracy, size, ease of use and portability.

Spirometry (meaning the measuring of breath) is the most common of the pulmonary function tests (PFTs), measuring lung function, specifically the amount (volume) and/or speed (flow) of air that can be inhaled and exhaled. Spirometry is an important tool used for generating pneumotachographs, which are helpful in assessing conditions such as asthma, pulmonary fibrosis, cystic fibrosis, and COPD.[3]

Procedure:

The basic forced volume vital capacity (FVC) test varies slightly depending on the equipment used. Generally, the subject is asked to take the deepest breath they can, and then exhale into the sensor as hard as possible, for as long as possible, preferably at least 6 seconds. It is sometimes directly followed by a rapid inhalation (inspiration), in particular when assessing possible upper airway obstruction. Sometimes, the test will be preceded by a period of quiet breathing in and out from the sensor (tidal volume), or the rapid breath in (forced inspiratory part) will come before the forced exhalation. During the test, soft nose clips may be used to prevent air escaping through the nose. Filter mouthpieces may be used to prevent the spread of microorganisms.

Pulmonary function tests can be used to:

- Compare your lung function with known standards that show how well your lungs should be working.

- Measure the effect of chronic diseases like asthma, chronic obstructive lung disease (COPD), or cystic fibrosis on lung function.

- Identify early changes in lung function that might show a need for a change in treatment.

- Detect narrowing in the airways.

- Decide if a medicine (such as a bronchodilator) could be helpful to use.

- Show whether exposure to substances in your home or workplace have harmed your lungs.

- Determine your ability to tolerate surgery and medical procedures

---

Check the spirometer calibration
Explain the test
Prepare the subject
　　Ask about smoking, recent illness, medication use, etc.
　　Measure weight and height without shoes
Wash hands
Instruct and demonstrate the test to the subject, to include
　　Correct posture with head slightly elevated
　　Inhale rapidly and completely
　　Position of the mouthpiece (open circuit)
　　Exhale with maximal force

Perform maneuvers (closed circuit method)

Have subject assume the correct posture

Attach nose clip, place mouthpiece in mouth and close lips around the mouthpiece

Inhale completely and rapidly with a pause of ,1 s at TLC

Exhale maximally until no more air can be expelled while maintaining an upright posture

Repeat instructions as necessary, coaching vigorously

Repeat for a minimum of three maneuvers; no more than eight are usually required

Check test repeatability and perform more maneuvers as necessary

Perform maneuver (open circuit method)

Have subject assume the correct posture

Attach nose clip

Inhale completely and rapidly with a pause of ,1 s at TLC

Place mouthpiece in mouth and close lips around the mouthpiece

Exhale maximally until no more air can be expelled while maintaining an upright posture

Repeat instructions as necessary, coaching vigorously

Repeat for a minimum of three maneuvers; no more than eight are usually required

Check test repeatability and perform more maneuvers as necessary

Table 2: Procedures for recording forced vital capacity

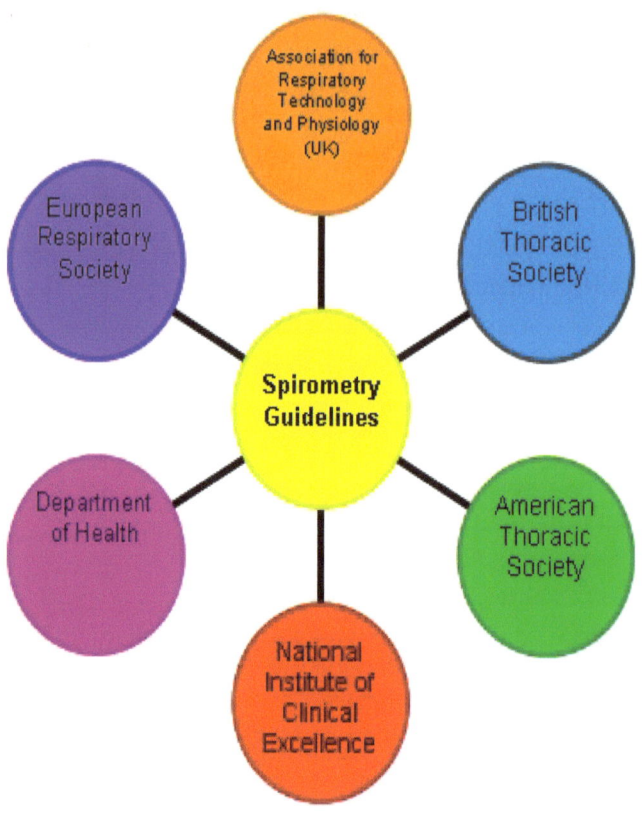

Picture 1: Guidelines for Spirometry

Limitations of test:

The maneuver is highly dependent on subject cooperation and effort, and is normally repeated at least three times to ensure reproducibility. Since results are dependent on subject cooperation, FVC can only be underestimated, never overestimated. Due to the subject cooperation required, Spirometry can only be used on children old enough to comprehend and follow the instructions given (6 years old or more), and only on subjects who are able to understand and follow instructions, thus this test is not suitable for subjects who are unconscious, heavily sedated, or have limitations that would interfere with vigorous respiratory efforts. Other types of lung function tests are available for infants and unconscious persons.

Another major limitation is the fact that many intermittent or mild asthmatics have normal Spirometry between acute exacerbations, limiting spirometry's usefulness as a diagnostic tool. It is more useful as a monitoring tool: a sudden decrease in FEV1 or other spirometric measures in the same patient can signal worsening control, even if the raw value is still normal. Subjects are encouraged to record their personal best measures.

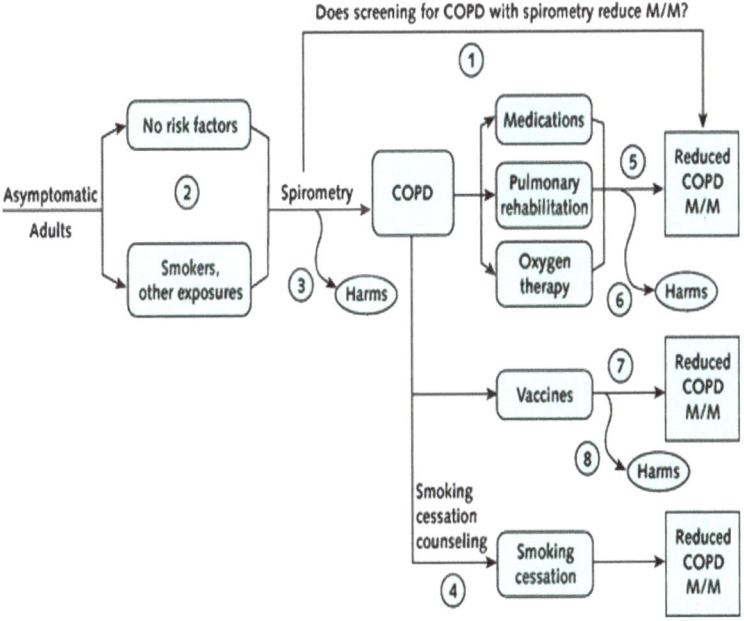

Picture 2: Limitations for Spirometry

Parameters:

The most common parameters measured in Spirometry are Vital capacity (VC), Forced vital capacity (FVC), Forced expiratory volume (FEV) at timed intervals of 0.5, 1.0 (FEV1), 2.0, and 3.0 seconds, forced expiratory flow 25–75% (FEF 25–75) and maximal voluntary ventilation (MVV)[4], also known as Maximum breathing capacity and other tests may be performed in certain situations[5].

Results are usually given in both raw data (litres, litres per second) and percent predicted. The test result as a percent of the "predicted values" for the patients of similar characteristics (height, age, sex, and sometimes race and weight). The interpretation of the results can vary depending on the physician and the source of the predicted values. Generally speaking, results nearest to 100% predicted are the most normal, and results over 80% are often considered normal.

Forced vital capacity (FVC):

Forced vital capacity (FVC) is the volume of air that can forcibly be blown out after full inspiration measured in liters. FVC is the most basic maneuver in Spirometry tests.[6]

Forced expiratory volume in 1 second (FEV1):

FEV1 is the volume of air that can forcibly be blown out in one second, after full inspiration.[6] Average values for FEV1 in healthy people depend mainly on sex and age, according to the diagram at left. Values of between 80% and 120% of the average value are considered normal.[7]

FEV1/FVC ratio (FEV1%):

FEV1/FVC (FEV1%) is the ratio of FEV1 to FVC. In healthy adults this should be approximately 75–80%. In obstructive diseases (asthma, COPD, chronic bronchitis, emphysema) FEV1 is diminished because of increased airway resistance to expiratory flow; the FVC may be decreased as well, due to the premature closure of airway in expiration, just not in the same proportion as FEV1 (for instance, both FEV1 and FVC are reduced, but the former is more affected because of the increased airway resistance). This generates a reduced value (<80%, often 45%). In restrictive diseases (such as pulmonary fibrosis) the FEV1 and FVC are both reduced proportionally and the value may be normal or even increased as a result of decreased lung compliance.

Forced expiratory flow (FEF):

Forced expiratory flow (FEF) is the flow (or speed) of air coming out of the lung during the middle portion of a forced expiration. It can be given at discrete times, generally defined by what fraction remains of the forced vital capacity (FVC). The usual intervals are 25%, 50% and 75% (FEF25, FEF50 and FEF75), or 25% and 50% of FVC. It can also be given as a mean of the flow during an interval, also generally delimited by when specific fractions remain of FVC, usually 25–75% (FEF25–75%). Average ranges in the healthy population depend mainly on sex and age, with FEF25–75% shown in diagram at left. Values ranging from 50-60%, and up to 130% of the average are considered normal.[7] MMEF or MEF stands for maximal (mid) expiratory flow and is the peak of expiratory flow as taken from the flow volume curve and measured in liters per second. It should theoretically be identical to peak expiratory flow (PEF), which is, however, generally measured by a peak flow meter and given in liters per minute.[8]

Forced inspiratory flow 25–75% or 25–50%:

Forced inspiratory flow 25–75% or 25–50% (FIF 25–75% or 25–50%) is similar to FEF 25–75% or 25–50% except the measurement is taken during inspiration.

Peak expiratory flow (PEF):

Peak expiratory flow (PEF) is the maximal flow (or speed) achieved during the maximally forced expiration initiated at full inspiration, measured in liters per minute or in liters per second.

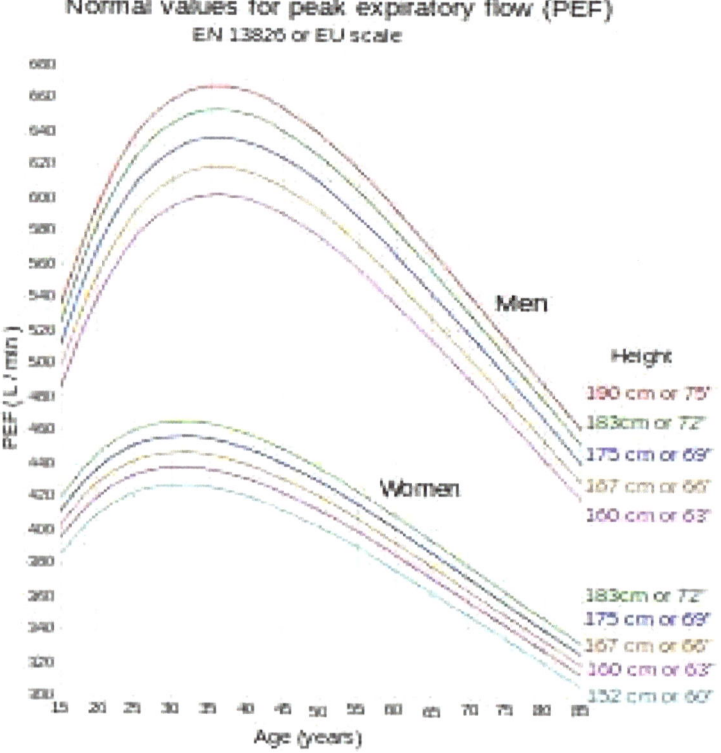

Picture 3: Normal values for peak expiratory flow (PEF), shown on EU scale.[9]

Tidal volume (TV):

Tidal volume is the amount of air inhaled and exhaled normally at rest.

Total lung capacity (TLC):

Total lung capacity (TLC) is the maximum volume of air present in the lungs.

Lung capacities and flow volumes:

Volume displacement spirometers can be bellows, pistons or bells over water which moves up and down as the subject breathes in and out of them. They can move a pen on a rotating drum to plot a chart of breathing volumes against time. Nowadays, electronic flow detection or turbine spirometers are replacing the older types. These produce computer generated charts of flow rates as well as volumes. For example, a spirometer can be used to find the vital capacity of the lungs.

Diffusing capacity (DLCO):

Diffusing capacity (or DLCO) is the carbon monoxide uptake from a single inspiration in a standard time (usually 10 sec). Since air consists of very minute or traces quantities of CO, 10 seconds is considered to be the standard time for inhalation, and then rapidly blow it out (exhale). The exhaled gas is tested to determine how much of the tracer gas was absorbed during the breath. This will pick up diffusion impairments, for instance in pulmonary fibrosis. This must be corrected for anemia (because rapid CO diffusion is dependent on hemoglobin in RBC's; a low hemoglobin concentration, anemia, will reduce DLCO) and pulmonary hemorrhage (excess RBC's in the interstitium or alveoli can absorb CO and artificially increase the DLCO capacity). Atmospheric pressure and/or altitude will also affect measured DLCO, and so a correction factor is needed to adjust for standard pressure.[10]

Maximum voluntary ventilation (MVV):

Maximum voluntary ventilation (MVV) is a measure of the maximum amount of air that can be inhaled and exhaled within one minute. For the comfort of the patient this is done over a 15 second time period before being extrapolated to a value for one minute expressed as liters/minute. Average values for males and females are 140–180 and 80–120 liters per minute respectively.

Critical Factors When Conducting Spirometry Testing Over Time

1. Standardize and document the testing protocol, equipment used, and all protocol or equipment changes.

2. Provide technicians with initial and periodic training, and periodically audit technical quality of Spirograms (QA reviews).

3. Maintain equipment
   - Avoid unneeded equipment changes.
   - Avoid unnecessary changes in spirometer configuration.
   - Verify spirometer accuracy.

a. Obtain evidence of validation testing of spirometer from the manufacturer

b. Check calibration at least daily during use

c. Routinely evaluate technical quality of Spirograms and patterns of test results

Save calibration records for as long as needed to support accuracy of Spirometry results.

4. Minimize biological variability
   - Conduct testing in same posture as previous tests (e.g., standing or sitting).
   - Conduct testing at the same time of day and season to assess long-term change.
   - Postpone testing for one hour after smoking, using a bronchodilator, or eating a heavy meal; three days after recovering from an illness that lasted three weeks or less; three weeks after a severe respiratory illness or ear infection; and six or more weeks after eye, ear, chest, or abdominal surgery, unless a surgeon provides a release statement.

Table 3: Critical Factors When Conducting Spirometry Testing Over Time.[11]

Spirometry results mean:

To determine whether a person has COPD, his or her Spirometry results are compared to normal or "predicted" values. The predicted values depend on a person's age, height, sex, and ethnicity. COPD obstructs and slows the flow of air into and out of the lungs. Therefore, in a person with COPD, both FEV1 and FEV1/FVC are lower than normal. According to the GOLD report, an FEV1/FVC ratio less than 0.7 means that a person is likely to have COPD. When COPD is present, the degree of reduction in FEV1, or degree of airflow limitation, is one indicator of the severity of the disease. According to the GOLD classification system, FEV1 at least 80% of the normal value indicates Mild airflow limitation, FEV1 between 50% and 80% of normal indicates Moderate airflow limitation, FEV1 between 30% and 50% of normal indicates Severe airflow limitation, and FEV1 below 30% of normal indicates Very Severe airflow limitation. A person's symptoms, history of exacerbations (periodic worsening of COPD symptoms), and other health problems also contribute to the overall severity of COPD.[11]

Basics of Respiration:

The respiratory tract consists of the trachea, lungs, bronchi, bronchioles, and alveoli. The alveoli constitute both the functional unit of the lung and the site of cellular respiration. From the trachea, the airways divide progressively like branching trees in both symmetrical and asymmetrical fashion: each branch of airways leading away from the trachea becomes smaller, but in turn the total area of cross-sectional airways actually increases. As a result, airflow resistance decreases as air moves from the large airways to the smaller bronchioles.

Bronchi, Bronchial Tree, and Lungs

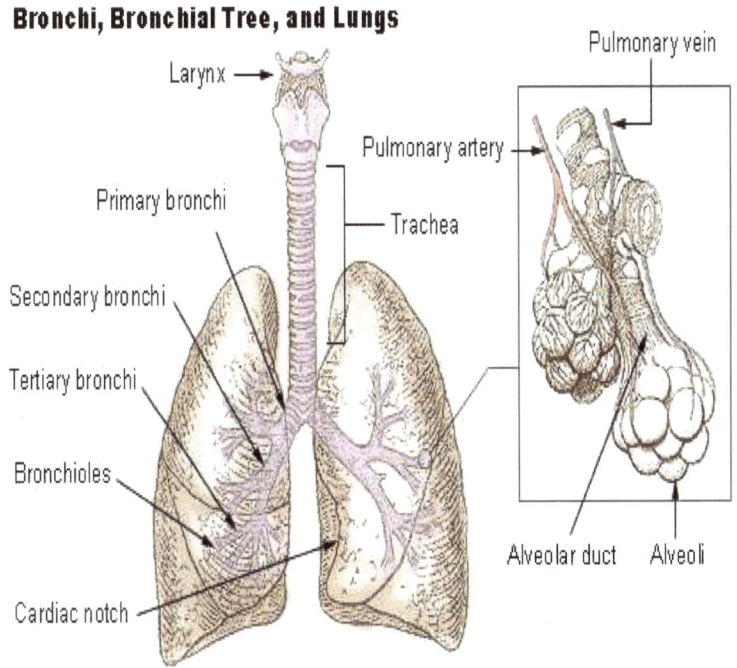

The movement of air in and out of the lungs is called ventilation that includes both inspiration and expiration. Inspiration, or inhalation, is an active process that utilizes muscles in the chest, primarily the diaphragm. Expiration, or exhalation, is normally a passive process that requires little muscular activity unless air is forcefully expelled from the lungs, such as during a forced vital capacity maneuver. The main purpose of the respiratory tract is to conduct air between the external environment and the surface of the alveoli to permit an exchange of oxygen and carbon dioxide.

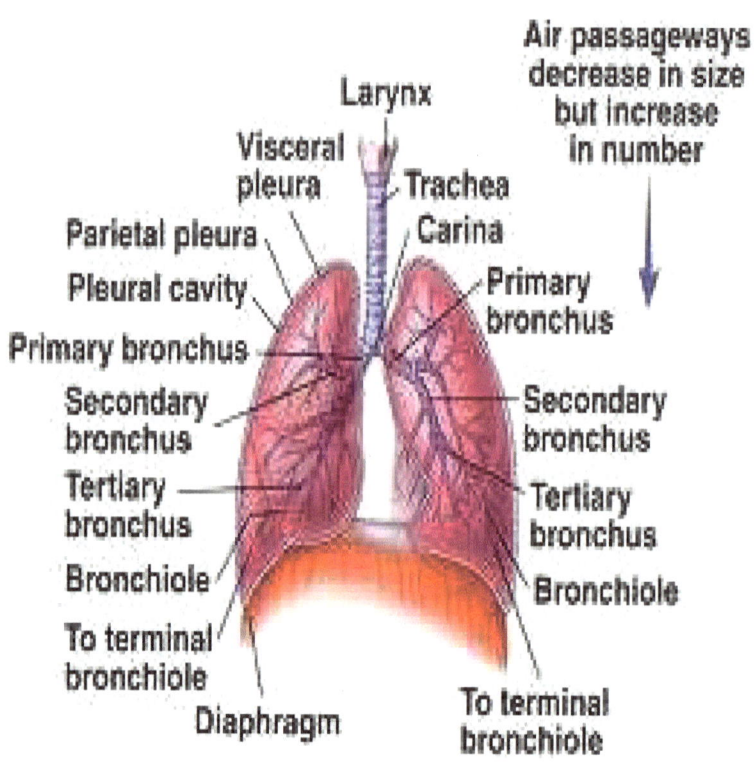

Air passageways decrease in size but increase in number

Larynx

Visceral pleura

Trachea

Parietal pleura

Carina

Pleural cavity

Primary bronchus

Primary bronchus

Secondary bronchus

Secondary bronchus

Tertiary bronchus

Tertiary bronchus

Bronchiole

Bronchiole

To terminal bronchiole

To terminal bronchiole

Diaphragm

The Respiratory tract

Spirometry testing does not directly measure the rate of oxygen transfer to the lungs; rather it measures lung volume and air flow rates, which are major factors that influence the process of oxygen transfer. The exchange of oxygen from the outside environment for carbon dioxide from venous blood defines the fundamental process of respiration. This exchange occurs at the surface of each of the approximately 300 million alveoli contained in the lungs. The alveoli have a combined total surface area for gas exchange that is equivalent to the size of a tennis court.[11,12]

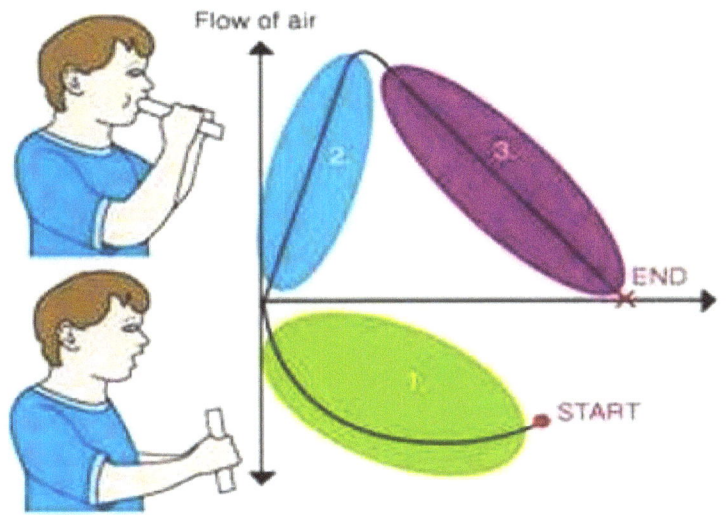

The lung is served by two blood supplies: pulmonary and bronchial. Pulmonary circulation pumps oxygen-depleted venous blood from the heart through the pulmonary arteries and to the lungs to be oxygenated before being pumped by the heart to the rest of the body. Bronchial circulation arises from the aorta (the largest artery coming from the heart) and pumps oxygenated blood to the lungs, providing the primary supply of blood for the lung tissue itself. Finally, while the main purpose is to facilitate the transfer of oxygen and carbon dioxide, the lung also serves other functions: metabolism and detoxification of a wide range of substances; protection against infectious agents and environmental pollutants; and the synthesis of important compounds such as prostaglandins, which are important in inflammatory reactions[12,13].

MIZAJ

Definition:

All types of bodies (animate and inanimate) which are found in this world, are formed by four *Ustaqissat* (elements) after mixing of with each other in different or in uniform quantities in accordance with the needs of the body. As a result of this mixing one quality dominates over the body, and this is called *Mizaj*.[14,15,16,17,18,19]

The literal meaning of Mizaj-

Mizaj, as Ibn Nafis describes, means intermixing of different components (Arkan) and is used as a noun instead of adjective.

Generally the word 'Temperament' is used as an English equivalent to Arabic term 'Mizaj'. The word temperament is derived from Latin word 'Tempero' meaning to mix or temper.[20]

Greeks would call the mixture of the humours as 'krasis' which is derived from 'kerannyni' i.e. to mix the word krasis is usually translated as temperament.[21]

The meanings of word 'temperament' as given in some dictionaries are mentioned below:

Temperament (L. temperamentum)- The physical organization peculiar to the individual including his character, or personality' predisposition, which influence his manner of thought and action, and general views of life.

(Illustrated Stedman's Medical dictionary, 24th Edition)

Temperament (L. temperamentum)- The combination of intellectual, emotional, ethical and physical characteristics of specific individual.

(Tabers Cyclopedic Medical Dictionary, 19th Edition).

Temperament (L.temperamentum)- the peculiar physical character and mental cast of an individual. **(Medical Dictionary by W.A. Newman).**

Temperament(L.temperamentum)- the mental, moral and emotional constitution, natural disposition, a violent passionate nature, the slightly inaccurate adjustment of the intervals on a key board instrument which makes it possible to play harmoniously in all keys.

(Odham's Medical Dictionary of English language).

According to Arab physicians, the word Mizaj is originated from the Arabic word "Imtezaj" which means the mixture of any humour (khilt) with any substance. As the Arabic word "Mizaj" denotes the idea of intermixture, so the mediaeval translators used the word commixtio or complexio which carry the meaning of mixing and weaving.

THE CONCEPT OF MIZAJ

Mizaj is one of the basic and fundamental concepts of Unani system of medicine and it is the most important part of Unani system of medicine. Our ancient Unani physicians were very much devoted towards the concept of Mizaj. The Arab era applied the concept of Mizaj on universal scale, but in the modern era the temperament is limited only for the psychosomatic dimensions. Mizaj is one of the basic and distinguishing features of unani medicine. It is one among the seven basic physiological principles (*Umoor-e-Tabiyah*). It forms the basis of pathology, diagnosis and treatment. Unani medicine's chief advantage over western medicine lies in its ability to provide a holistic treatment. Unani system of medicine provides this holism by mean of Mizaj.

The concept of Mizaj, is a major pillar of Tibb philosophy, is the amalgam of a person's physical characteristics and his /her psychological and emotional attributes. [22]

DEFINITION OF MIZAJ

Several Unani physicians have explained the definition of Mizaj according to their conceptual views. It is presented here in chronological order.

Majoosi defined the *Mizaj* as "all sorts of bodies (light or heavy), which are found in this ever-changing world, are formed by four elements (*ustuqussat*) after mixing in different or uniform quantities in accordance with the needs (of the body). As a result of this mixing, one or two qualities become dominant over the body, and this is called Mizaj. It is derived from Arabic word Imtizaj meaning to mix with each other". [21,23]

Masihi defined the *Mizaj* as "because there are so many primary components (*ustuqussat*) of the body, which are mixed together not in close proximity. Thus it is necessary that the qualities of primary compounds must be mixed as a whole. New qualities arises from intermixing of primary components which will be in between the previous qualities called Mizaj". [24,25]

Ibn Sina defined the *Mizaj* as "*Mizaj* is a quality which is produced by the action and reaction of different qualities of such type of elements which are divided in small particles so that the maximum particles of each element can be mixed as a whole. So when these small particles mix in each other by their properties, they act and react, resulting in generation of a new property (quality) which is equally found in the different particles of elements. This new quality is known as Mizaj." [26]

Ismail Jurjani defined the *Mizaj* as "when different qualities of elements acts and reacts by their powers then

36

previous qualities become diminished and a new moderate quality is developed which is known as *Mizaj*." [27]

Ali Ibn Habal Baghdadi defined the *Mizaj* as "when small elements get admixture, most of the particles of elements mix with each other and their various qualities act and react so heat overcomes the cold and cold overcomes the heat, similarly dryness overcomes the wetness and wetness overcomes the dryness and low grade qualities, light weight particles mix with high weight particles until a new quality is developed which is equally found in all the components of elements, this new moderate quality is known as Mizaj ." [28]

Allama Nafis defined the mizaj as "when after dividing in smaller particles the element mix with each other, they act and reacts which results in developing a new moderate quality in between the all four previous qualities, this new moderate quality is known as mizaj".[29]

Daood Antaqi defined as "Mizaj is a uniform quality which originates by the action and reaction of four elements, which are divided in smaller particles, so that the maximum particles of each can mix with each other".[30]

Hakim Mohd. Iliyas Khan defined the Mizaj as "Mizaj is such type of moderate quality, which is produced by the action and reaction and chemical changes in the small particles of different elements, which occur due to the effects of their specific powers. This moderate quality may be differing in different persons and in different species also".[31]

Gruner defined as "temperament is that quality which result from the mutual interaction and interspersion of the four contrary primary qualities residing within the (imponderable) elements". These elements are so minutely intermingled as each to lie in very intimate relationship to one another. Their opposite powers alternatively conquered until a state of equilibrium is reached which is uniform throughout the whole. It is this outcome that is called "the temperament".[32]

Abdul Latif Falsafi defined the Mizaj as "when smaller particles of different elements join each other in such a way that the particles of each elements mix with the particles of other elements, it results in breakdown of qualities of all elements, due to which the qualities of the total particles converted into a moderate quality. This moderate quality is known as Mizaj which dissociates in all the particles".[33]

Ayyub Israili defined Mizaj as "Mizaj is such type of moderate quality which is originated by the action and reaction of different opposite qualities. When four elements mix with each other and one element effects the other then they break to small particles due to action and reaction process. This process should be of such type that the biochemical structure of each element breaks the strength of quality of other elements, resulting in generation of a moderate secondary quality. This moderate secondary quality is known as mizaj".[34]

Allama Sadidi described as "*Mizaj* is such type of *Malmoosa* (touching) quality which is produced by effect of different qualities of smaller particles of elements and the character to adopt the effects of these different qualities".[35]

Hkm. Latif writes as the word **'temperament'** is metaphorically applied to the admixed state of such a compound, because it is due to this admixture that such an admixed state is produced. Therefore temperament is the one name given both to the cause and effect".[36]

Shah writes that **"temperament** is the pattern of qualities as a whole which emerges from the action and reaction of the mass and energy and thus in the human organism of the structure and functions. As the basic qualities of the energy are heat and cold and the mass, dryness and moisture their natural interactions lead to the emergence of a new balance of qualities which varies with the quantitative proportion of the primary qualities".[37]

Mehdi Hasan describes the temperament along with the four elements. He says that "the four elements are the resultant of four qualities moisture, cold, dryness and heat. Two qualities go to constitute an element thus;

Heat+Moisture = Air

Cold+Moisture = Water

The ultimate units are pure qualities. These have been identified as follows:

Heat = Oxidation

Cold = Reduction

Moisture = Hydration

Dryness = Dehydration

In this aspect temperament can be understood by the following example as

Saudavi or melancholic temperament should be interpreted not as cold &dry but in which reduction and dehydration are preponderating.[38]

Hkm Sayed Ishtiyaq Ahmad described the *Mizaj* as "*Mizaj* is defined as the new state of a matter, having quality, different from the present in the elements or compounds before coming into Imtizaj (intermixture of chemical combination), which results from the action and reaction of the contrary

39

qualities and powers, present in the minute particles (atoms) of different elements (or molecules of different compounds) when they are combined together, the resultant new quality, a uniform state on the state of equilibrium emerging after the combination of more than one elements is called Mizaj".[39]

Tayyab suggest in "Greece Arab Medicine", that the temperament is synthetic concepts which express the various physical as well as psychological tendencies of the individual in terms of matter and energy i.e. activity as heat and cold reactivity as dryness and moisture".[40]

Altaf Ahmad Azmi defines the temperament as "temperament means final combination or form of elements. In the other words, formation of temperament in a compound depends on the, number, ratio and atomic sequence of element in the compound. The properties created in the compound differ from the properties of its constituents. A compound retains its properties so long as its elemental form is held together".[21]

Zaidi and Zulkifle describe the temperament as "Temperament is an intrinsic state, which enables an individual to survive and to procreate comfortably and is responsible for distinctive morpho-bio-physio-immuno-psychological identity of the individual".[25]

By above described views of eminent *Unani* scholars it is evident that Mizaj is a new state which is the result of the actions and reactions between the contrary qualities, present in different elements. On the other hand we can say that the resultant uniform state which emerges after the combination of the properties of more than one element is called Mizaj, which makes every compound differ in nature. For the formation of temperament it is necessary that different elements get combined together and form a new compound .In *Unani Tibb* the process of formation of new compound by intermixing of different elements is termed as *Imtizaj.*

Types:

If a compound is formed by the interaction of four elements with their equal quantities, a *kafiat* (quality) is produced in the compound which is known as *Mizaje mo'tadil* (equable temperament). And if a compound is formed after mixing of four elements with their unequal quantities, a quality produced in the compound, it will be *Mizaj* (temperament) of the compound. For example, if the dominant element (part) in the compound is *Nar* (fire), the compound would be considered as of *Har Mizaj* (hot temperament). Similarly, if the dominant element or part of the compound is *Maa* (water), the compound would be considered as of *Barid Mizaj* (cold temperament) and if, the dominant part of the compound is *Hawa* (air) that is called as of *Ratab Mizaj* (moist temperament). And if the dominant part or element in the compound is *Arz* (soil), the compound would be called as of *Yabis Mizaj* (dry temperament).

Similarly, if two elements out of four *Ustaqissat* (fire, air, water, soil) become dominant, the compound would be called by their names. For example, if fire and air both are dominant in the compound, it would be considered as *Har Ratab*. Likewise there are four types *of* *Murakkab Mizaj* as *Har Ratab, Har Yabis, Barid Ratab* and *Barid Yabis.* [14,15,16,17,18,19]
Thus there are 9 types of *Mizaj* , one is *Mo'tadil* and eight are *Ghair Mo'tadil (Tibbi Mo'tadil).* [14,15,16,17,18,19]

Because of intermixing of elements in different proportion in the compounds, numbers of *Mizaj* may exceed the 9 and can reach beyond the limit of counting. That's why each individual has its specific *Mizaj.* [16]

***Mizaj* of the organs:**

Every species is created with its specific *Mizaj* which is beneficial and suitable for the same. This is the temperament which is known as ***Mizaje Mo'tadil (Tibbi mu'tadil)*** for it. For example, a lion has more heat (hot temperament) than other animals so that it may get more anger and may attack easily on his prey (***Shikar***) for diet. Similarly, a rabbit has been created with cold temperament so that it may get more fear from other animals and easily go away for saving his life. This is nothing but it is only for his benefit and requirements. Similarly different organs of the body have been provided different types of *Mizaj* as per their functional requirements. For example, there are some organs of ***Mizaje Mo'tadil*** e.g. skin. Some organs are of hot temperament. Some are of moist and some others are of dry and the few are of cold temperament. The organs having hot temperament are in descending order; heart, liver, meat (muscles), spleen, kidneys, arteries and vessels. The organs having cold temperament are in decreasing order like hair, bones, cartilages, ligaments, tendons, membranes, spinal cord, brain and fats.

The organs having moist temperament are in decreasing order as ***Samin*** (type of fats), ***Shahm***, brain, breast, testes, lungs, liver, spleen, kidney, muscles. The organs having dry temperament are in descending order as hair, bones, cartilage, ligament, tendon, membranes, arteries, vessels, motor nerve, heart and sensory nerves.

These organ's temperaments are known as *Eitidale Tibbi* for them. [14,15,16,17,18]

***Akhlat* and its Temperament:**

Akhlat are the things liquid in nature, formed from the diet when it gets metabolized firstly in the liver. All organs of the body are formed from the ***Akhlat***. *Akhlat* are of 4 types i.e.; blood, phlegm, bile and black bile.

- Temperament of **Dam** (blood) is *Har Ratab.*
- Temperament of **Balgham** (phlegm) is *Barid Ratab.*
- Temperament of **Safra** (bile) is *Har Yabis.*

Temperament of **Sauda** (black bile) is *Barid Yabis.*
14,15,16,17,18,41,42.43,44,45

TEMPERAMENT OF ASNAN (AGES):

Whole life of the human being has been divided into 4 stages i.e. *Sinne Numoo, Sinne Shabab, Sinne Kuhoolat and Sinne Shaikhookhat.*
- Temperament of **Sinne Numoo** is *Har Ratab.*
- Temperament of **Sinne Shabab** is *Har Yabis.*
- Temperament of **Sinne Kuhoolat** is *Barid Yabis.*
- Temperament of **Sinne Shaikhookhat** is *Barid Yabis* (extremely). [15,16,17,18]

Temperament of *Mausam* (seasson):
- *Mizaj* of *Mausame Rabi* is *Mo'tadil.*
- *Mizaj* of *Mausame Saif* is *Har Yabis.*
- *Mizaj* of *Mausame Kharif* is *Barid Yabis* (*Yubusat > Burudat*).
- Mizaj of *Mausame Sarma* is *Barid Ratab* (*Burudat > Rutubat*). [15,16]

Temperament of *Ajnas* (sexes):
- Temperament of male is *Har Ratab.*
- Temperament of female is *Barid Ratab* as compared to male. [15,16]

Types of *Mizaje Mo'tadil Tibbi* according to Species, Races, Persons and Organs:

The *Mizaj* can be divided into 8 kinds as per species, races, persons and organs of the body as:
- *Mizaje Mo'tadil Nau'ee bil Qiyas elal Kharij* (Equable temperament of a species as a whole):

This temperament distinguishes a species as a whole from the other. This temperament of a species is most benefitting and

43

suitable for that species (human being) and not suitable and not benefitting for other species (like animals).

- *Mizaje Mo'tadil Nau'ee bil Qiyas elal Dakhil* (Most equable temperament of a member of the species):
- *Mizaje Mo'tadil Sinfi bil Qiyas elal Kharij* (Equable temperament of a race as compared to other races of a species):

  It depends upon the climatic and geographical condition of a country. For example, Indians and Africans have their specific temperament due to different geographical conditions.
- *Mizaje Mo'tadil Sinfi bil Qiyas elal Dakhil* (Most equable temperament of a member of a race as compared to other members of the same race of a species):
- *Mizaje Mo'tadil Shakhsi bil Qiyas elal Kharij* (Equable temperament of a person of a race):

  It is the most suitable temperament for the normal functioning of the body of an individual as compared to others.
- *Mizaje Mo'tadil Shakhsi bil Qiyas elal Dakhil* (Equable temperament of a person as compared to his own temperament in different states): For example, the *Mizaj* achieved in youth or in *Rabi* season by a person will be more suitable than that of other states of life and season.
- *Mizaje Mo'tadil Uzwi bil Qiyas elal Kharij* (Equable temperament of an organ as compared to other organs of the body):

  This temperament of an organ is most benefitting and suitable for the same.
- *Mizaje Mo'tadil Uzwi bil Qiyas elal Dakhil* (Equable temperament of an organ by physiological functional state):

  This temperament is achieved by an organ when it is performing its functions with full efficiency.[15,16]

Types of *Sue Mizaj* (*Mizaje Ghair Mo'tadil*)**:**
When a *Kaifiyat* (quality) is increased from *E'tidal* (balance) the condition is known as "*Mizaje Ghair Mo'tadil*" or *Sue Mizaj*.

Sue Mizaj **is of 2 types:**
- *Sue Mizaj Sada* (simple imbalance temperament without matter)
- *Sue Mizaj Maddi* (imbalance temperament due to any matter)

Sue Mizaj Sada **is of 2 types:**
- **Sue Mizaj Mufrad Sada**: When one *Kaifiyat* out of *Kaifiate Arbaa* is increased in any compound, it is known as *Sue Mizaj Mufrad Sada*. It is of 4 types.
- **Sue Mizaj Murakkab Sada**: When *Mizaj* is deviated in 2 *Kaifiyat* (qualities) out of *Kaifiyate Arba* then it is known as *Sue Mizaj Murakkab Sada*. It is also of 4 types.

Sue Mizaj Maddi **is of 2 types**:
- **Sue Mizaj Mufrad Maddi** (single-imbalance temperament due to any matter): *Sue Mizaj Mufrad Maddi* is the temperament in which one *kaifiyat* dominated substance(s) is increased. It is of 4 types.
- **Sue Mizaj Murakkab Maddi** (compound imbalance temperament due to any matter): It is the temperament in which 2 *Kaifiyat* dominated substance(s) increased. It is also of 4 types.

Like this, there are 16 types of *Sue Mizaj* as:
- **Sue Mizaj Mufrad Sada**: *Har, Barid, Ratab* and *Yabis*.
- **Sue Mizaj Murakkab Sada**: *Har Ratab, Har Yabis, Barid Ratab, Barid Yabis*.
- **Sue Mizaj Mufrad Maddi**: *Har Maddi, Barid Maddi, Ratab Maddi, Yabis Maddi*.

- *Sue Mizaj Murakkab Maddi*: *Har Ratab Maddi, Har Yabis Maddi, Barid Ratab Maddi, Barid Yabis Maddi.*[15]

The modulators or factors responsible for changing the temperament of human being are of 2 types:

- Internal Factors (Internal environmental factors).
- External factors (External environmental factors).[15,16]
- **Internal Factors (Internal environmental factors):**

   These are the factors which influence the temperament of human being at the time of its formation and development in the uterus. The foetal development is the outcome of interaction between the gamets (sperm and ova) of the parents. Gamets, undoubtedly, transfer parental characters to the offspring. *Unani* physicians are of the opinion that some active forces (*Quwwate Mughayyirae Oola and Musawwirah*) in utero, determine the morphological and biochemical composition of the foetus in the light of temperament of the gamets.

   Any abnormal change in the *Maaddae Manwiah* (gamets) may alter the temperament of the foetus because of which different types of congenital deformities are developed in the foetus. For example, if the semen or gamets is less or more in quantity, foetus will not be developed properly. If *Maddae Manwiah* is less in quantity any organ maybe smaller in size as in "Microcephaly". Similarly, if the quantity of *Mani* is more, any organ of the body may enlarge as in "Macrocephally."[15,16]

There are so many kinds of congenital diseases that develop in child due to any disturbance in the genetic material (chromosomes and genes) in the uterus like,

- Congenital rubella syndrome[46]
- Down's syndrome[46,47,48,49,50,51]

- Thelassimia[52]
- PKU (phenylketonurea)[47,53]

Till now, over 2300 hereditary diseases have been identified.[46]

2. External Environmental Factors:

These include

Age, Air, Season, Habitat (Residence), Occupation and Habits.

Age: Age of an individual is the factor which influences the temperament directly. Every person has specific temperament in different phases of life which is responsible for health and diseases of an individual. Because of abnormal changes in this temperament, so many diseases may develop in the body.[14,15,54]

Air (Wind): It is one of the most important external environmental factors, responsible for influencing temperament of an individual. Although there are so many kinds of winds blow in the atmosphere, but, only four winds i.e. Northerly (cold dry), Southerly (hot moist), Easterly (equable temperament) and Westerly (cold dry or near to equable) are of great importance from medical point of view. Because of having their specific *Mizaj,* each wind is suitable for the person having opposite *Mizaj* and harmful or not suitable for the persons having same temperament as that of the wind and may cause diseases in the body accordingly. Northerly wind having cold dry temperament may cause diseases having cold dry temperament. Same like this, remaining winds tend to develop the diseases having same temperament as that of the winds.[14,15,54]

Season: It is also an important factor which may affect the temperament of human being. There are four types of seasons in the year. Each season has its specific *Mizaj* because of which it affects the temperament of an individual. If the temperament of human being and season become same, diseases having same temperament as that of the season and of human being may be developed. That's why; Dam (blood) related diseases occur in **Rabi,'** diseases related to *Safra* develop in the **Saif (Summer)** and diseases related to *Sauda* prevail in the **Kharif,** while

47

Balghami diseases occur in the **Winter** season. The diseases occurring in the end and in the beginning of the season are related with both pre and proceeding season.[14,15,54]

Habitat (residence/country/city): Habitat of an inhabitant exerts its effect directly on human life by its specific temperament. For example, Northern countries with cold and dry temperament, Southern countries with hot and moist, Eastern countries with *Mo'tadil* temperament and Western countries with *Mo'tadil mail ba Rutoobat* (moderately tilted toward *rutoobat*) which is similar to the temperament of *Mosame Kharif.* Because of specific *Mizaj* (temperament/ climate) of habitat, some specific diseases, related to the temperament of the same, are developed. [14,15.] For example, Inhabitants of hot places are generally of soft and delicate constitution of body, complexion of the body and hair are black. Similarly, inhabitants of cold places are usually strong and brave because, in cold temperament *Hararate Ghariziah* resides inside the body resulting in good digestion of inhabitants. If the temperament of these countries becomes damp or moist along with cold, persons living in these countries will become fleshy and fatty with inconspicuous veins (invisible).[14,15]

Inhabitants of damp countries are distinctly fleshy and fatty with soft and smooth skin.[14,15]

In dry countries, both winter and summer seasons are in their extreme condition, because of which temperaments of inhabitants of these places become dry, as a result their skin becomes rough and cracked. Their brain tends to be dry, because of which so many abnormal consequences may develop in the form of diseases.[14,15]

Residents of high altitudes are generally brave, strong and long lived. It is because of pure air having cold temperament which is present at these places.

Temperament of inhabitants of low land area is hot because of accumulation of hot air and hot water in these places. This atmosphere may predispose to some abnormalities in the inhabitants like,

- People are generally weak
- Infectious diseases are frequent
- People are of short stature with black hair.[14,15]

Inhabitants of *Masakine Hajariah Makshoofah* (stony soil uncovered with snow) Inhabitants of these places are more susceptible to develop some changes in the body like:

- They are of solid and hard body
- Because of dominance of *Yuboosat* on the body, their sleep is decreased
- Body is full of hair
- They are strong but their characters are bad
- They are active and intelligent in their work.[14,15]

Inhabitants of snow capped mountains are like those of cold countries. During snow fall these places are generally breezy because of fine air. After snow fall or when ice melts, the air causes suffocation here.[14,15]

Temperament of inhabitants of the cities or countries situated at the sea level:

Temperament of these inhabitants is *Mo'tadil Mail Ba Rutubat* because sea air is neither cold nor hot, therefore, *rutoobat* in the places becomes dominant.[14,15]

If residence is in North side, lowness or low level of ground and the vicinity of sea, it will make inhabitants of these countries more temperate and if residence is in southern countries temperament of residents will not be temperate.[14,15]

Habit is also an important factor to change the temperament of human being:

If a person adopts a habit for a long period, it will act like a *Mizaje Taba'i* for him, because *Aadat* (habit) considered as *Tabia'te Saniah*.

49

Aadat (Habit) of a person may be of so many kinds; for example, the person who is habitual to work in heat or hot environment like Black smith or the people who work before heat and fire in a factory or other places do not get trouble from heat, but when they go to the cold places or come in contact of cold air they will be affected from cold temperament or environment.

These people are more prone to develop hot diseases and have more capability to tolerate the heat.

Similarly, inhabitants of northern countries and the people whose occupation is related to water like fisherman, washer man, sailor etc. are not affected by cold temperament. These people are more susceptible to develop cold diseases in comparison to hot diseases. These diseases may be treated easily because the temperament of the diseases is similar to the temperament of the body.

Besides these two examples there are so many types of habits found in persons for example,

- Habit of eating of cold and hot food
- Habit of eating at specific time
- Habit of bathing
- Habit of sleep and wakefulness
- Habit of coitus.
- Habit of *Istifragh* (elimination) etc.[14,15]

Occupation: It is an important external environmental factor responsible for influencing the *Mizaj* of a person. For example, if a person is involved in such occupation in which he has to face heat or fire; in this condition he develops dryness (*Mizaje Yabis*) in his body because of which he will be more prone to develop dry diseases.

Similarly, if a person adopts such profession in which *buroodat* and *rutoobat* are in excess amount like fishery, sailing, washing of clothes etc, he will be more susceptible to develop diseases of cold and moist temperament.[14,15]

Sue Mizaj and consequences:

In Unani system of medicine, regarding temperament, there are some important principles by which we can predict or aware about the health of a person. For examples;

- If a person gets *Mizaje Asli* (congenital temperament) as *Har Yabis*, he will pass his whole life like an adult person.[55]
- If a person has such *Mizaje Asli* (furnished to him from mother) which has been deviated towards coldness (*buroodat*) or moistness, he will pass his life like an old person.[55]
- When a person having a specific *Mizaje Asli*, reaches the age that temperament is the same as that of the person, he will be disturbed and may fall ill. For example, a person having *Mizaje Asli* as hot dry, he will get difficulty when he reaches adulthood because of the same *Mizaj* of both, age and *Mizaje Asli*.[55]
- If a person having a *Mizaje Asli* as *Barid Ratab*, when he reaches adulthood, his temperament will be equable (*Mo'tadil*) because of Hot-dry temperament of adult hood and person will feel better and healthy.[55]
- If a person having hot moist temperament he will pass his life in better way when he reaches in middle age (*Sinne Kahoolat*) because of cold dry temperament of this age. In this age *Mizaj* of the person will be equable due to opposite temperament of age and *asli*.[55]
- If a person having a *Mizaje Har* and adopts hot *Tadabeeer* like hot diets, occupation, residence and season, he will get trouble surely and may involve in hot diseases.

51

Similarly, we can predict about the condition (health and disease) of the person having different types of *Mizaj* like, cold moist, or dry temperament or their combination.[15,55,]

- The persons of *Mo'tadil Mizaj* are more susceptible to *Khilti* diseases.
- The persons with Har Mizaj are to develop fever frequently.[17]

Determination of temperament:

Since structures and functions of organs and persons, as a whole, are determined by their respective temperaments. The physiological functions and variations thereof are used as means to determine *Mizaj* of an individual or of an organ.[15,16,56,57,58,59]

Different organs have their own specific temperaments which put together influence the temperaments of an individual, as a whole. Therefore temperament of an individual is the resultant of the temperament of all the organs. All individuals vary in their own temperament because of the variations in the temperament of their similar organs.

The determination of temperament is thus based on the signs and symptoms, which reflect the temperament of an individual most exponentially. According to the eminent Unani physicians like**, Majoosi** and **Jurjani**, determinants of temperament are 5 in number while **Ibn Sina** gave 10 determinants to assess the temperament of an individual or of an organ.

Now, these 10 determinants, are usually used to assess the temperament by physicians which are the following

- *Malmas* (**palpation**):

The state of warmth and coldness could be determined by touch. Similarly, roughness, firmness and softness of the skin and its appendages, especially nails could also be felt by palpation that indicates *Rutoobat* and *Yaboosat* of the body.

- *Lahm wa Shahm* (**flesh & fat**):

Excessive musculature indicates hot and moist temperament whereas excess quantity of fat is attributed to cold and moist one.

- *Sha'r* (**hair**):

To draw a conclusion about *Mizaj* from the state of hair is well pronounced.

Different states of hair are seen as:

- The higher rate of growth of the hair indicates hot dry temperament whereas it is decreased in cold temperament.
- Black dark colour of hair suggests hot temperament whereas reddish color is associated with "*Mo'tadil* "temperament.
- Coarse hair is generally found in hot temperament.
- Coarse and straight hairs are generally found in hot and moist temperament.
- Coarse and curly hair is found in hot dry temperament. Fine and scanty hair are present in the people having cold and dry temperament.
- Wide and dense distribution of hair on the chest indicates higher degree of hot temperament of the heart.
- Wide distribution of hair all over the body in general (extremities & trunk) is suggestive of hot temperament of the body.

- *Laune badan* (**complexion of the body**):

Reddish colour of the body is indicative of *Har Mizaj*. Whitish colour of the body indicates cold temperament where as yellowness of the body indicates hot dry temperament.

- *Haiyate Aa'za* (**physique**):

The morphological features of organs are indicative of their respective temperaments e.g. broad chest, prominence of veins and joints, well developed muscles, rapid and strong pulse, larger extremities and height of an individual all are indicative of hot temperament.

Narrow and small chest, inconspicuous veins, hidden joints, short stature, short extremities, slow and weak pulse and excessive fat deposition are the signs of cold temperament.

Since heat is a driving factor for various purposeful activities and development of the organs and parts of the body, so well developed organs or parts and increased physiological functions or activities of the body are indicative of hot temperament.

- *Kaifiate infe'al* (**responsiveness of organs/ Aa'za ka mutassir hona):**

    Each person's body or organs get affected by *Kafiate Arbaa* like *Hararat, Burudat, Rutoobat* and *Yaboosat* as per their temperaments furnished to them from mother.

    A person having cold temperament will be more influenced by coldness as compared to hot temperament. Similarly, if a person having hot temperament he is more influenced by heat. He feels hot, even, if there is a little bit excess in amount of heat in the environment. Similarly, persons having *Ratab Yabis Mizaj* can be imagined or understood.

- *Naum wa Yaqza* **(sleep and wakefulness):**

    Excess of sleep indicates preponderance of *Rutoobat* (fluid) and *Buroodat* (cold). Similarly, wakefulness beyond normal duration is indicative of *Mizaj Yabis* of the body (especially of brain).

- **Afaa'le Aa'za (functions of the organs):**

    Functions of the organs reflect their functional and structural integrity. An increase or acceleration in the functions and actions of the body beyond the physiological limit is an indication of hot temperament of the body. For example rapid growth of the body nails and hair is an indication of hot temperament.

- *Fuzlate badan*(excretae):

    There are some types of *fuzlate badan* like, urine, faeces, sweat and nasal secretion, excreted out from the body.

If these are being excreted out properly from the body of a person, it will be indication of *Mo'tadil Mizaj* of the same. And if these are not excreted out in right way, it will be an indication of *Sue Mizaj* of the body. For example, a person is excreting more sweat with pungent /bad odour; it will be indication of hot temperament of the same.

Similarly, if a person having semi solid faeces with pungent odour, it will indicate the hot temperament of the same.

- *Infe a'alate Nafsaniah* (**State of psyche**):

There are so many emotional states/ reflexes which are indicative of the temperament. These reflexes include mainly anger, anguish, feeling of sorrow, velar, activeness, decisiveness, well mannerism, considerations. All these indicate hot temperament. If these emotional reflexes persist beyond a reasonable limit, it will be an indication of dryness in the temperament (*Sue Mizaj Yabis*) in addition to heat. [15,16,56,57,58]

METHODOLOGY

Normal healthy individuals for present study were selected, from Ayurvedic and Unani Tibbia College, Karol Bagh, New Delhi for conducting the study of pulmonary functions pattern in the subjects in respect of their temperament. The individuals were selected on the basis of following criteria.

Inclusion Criteria:
1. Individuals of 18 to 30 years of age
2. Both sexes

Exclusion Criteria:
1. Person suffering from any disease
2. Person of age less than 18 years
3. Person of age more than 30 years

All the persons from A & U Tibbia College, New Delhi fulfilling the inclusion criteria were selected.

Parameters:

The objective parameters described in literature and quoted in review were assessed to determine the *Mizaj*. In addition two arbitrary parameters were devised to assess the *Mizaj i.e.* counting of hair in 1 inch squire area over the sternum and skin fold thickness. Besides, other subjective as well as objective parameters were assessed and observed carefully in every person. Some were based on *A'lamat Ajnase A'shra* (10 determinents) like *Malmas, Lah'am wa Shah'am, Sha'r (hair), Laune Badan, Haiate Aa'za, Kaifiate Aa'za, Naum wa Yqza, Afa'all Aa'za, Fuzlate Badan, Infia'alate Nafsaniah*. Regarding each *Alamat* all persons were observed and questioned about the things related to *Mizaj*. For example skin of the patients or subjects was palpated with dorsal aspect of the hand to assess hardness and softness of skin of the body for determining the amount of *Rutoobate Badan* (body fluids) to know *Mizaj* of the subject *i.e.* if *Malmas* (touch/ tactile) was soft, that means body

56

containing more or excess of fluid because of which body's temperament was considered tilted towards *Mizaj Ratab* and if *Malmas* was hard or dry that means *Rutoobat Badan* are diminished and *Mizaj* of the patient was going towards *Yaboosat*. Lastly on the basis of the total score of the 10 independent determinants, and signs and symptoms of dominance of *Akhlat*, a particular *Mizaj* was assigned to the person (Annexure 1).

Study Design: Observational study for the assessment of *Mizaj* and its correlation with pulmonary functions.

Sample size: 100 subjects

Duration : 6 Months.

Procedure of Study:

The subject fulfilling the inclusion criteria were selected, then their temperament was assessed by two prestructured proforma designed for the assessment of *Mizaj*. These were based on *A'lamat Ajnase A'shra* and *Ghalbae Akhlat* (Symptoms of dominance of humour of the body) respectively and pulmonary function test by spirometry.

After assessment of *Mizaj*, pulmonary functions relation in respect of *Mizaj* of the person was evaluated. Then appropriate *tadabeer* or guidelines, as a preventive measures, were advised to each and every subject individually, so that he may be aware about his health and the diseases for which he was more prone to develop in future.

Socioeconomic status (SES):

The SES was assesses by using the Kuppuswami's SES Scale for Urban population, 1976. Due to changes in the economy to year, the classification or scale was modified accordingly. The latest SES scale is of 2007 (Annexure No.2).

Height:

The height of individual was measured using a 200cm Stature Meter manufactured by BIOCON. The individual with bare foot were made to stand on a flat floor with feet parallel and with heels, shoulders and back of head touching the wall. The head was kept erect so that the orbit was in the same horizontal plane as the external auditory meatus. The scale then was brought down making a firm contact with vertex and was parallel to the floor, reading were recorded to the nearest of 0.5cm.

Weight:

The weight was measured in kilograms using electronic digital weighing machine to the nearest measure of 0.1 kg.

Body mass index or Quetelet's index:

The BMI was calculated using the formula mentioned below:

$$BMI = \frac{\text{Body weight in (Kg)}}{\text{height (m)}^2}$$

Data analysis:

Data were tabulated in a systematic way for presentation and analysis on the basis of recorded parameter regarding demographic profile.

Documentation:

Record has been submitted to the department of Munafe ul Aza, A & U Tibbia college, Karol Bagh, New Delhi

OBSERVATION AND RESULTS

Table No. 1

Distribution of the young adults according to Sex

(n=100)

Sex	No. of Patients	Percentage (%)
Male	67	67
Female	33	33
Total	**100**	**100%**

Figure No. 1

Distribution of young adults according to Sex

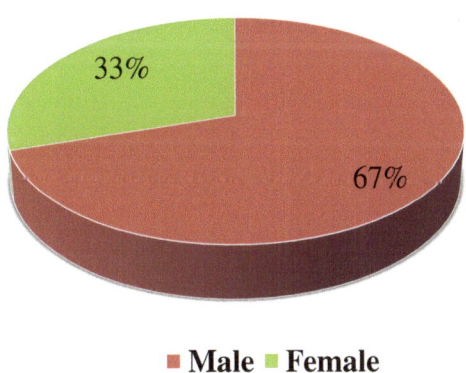

■ **Male** ■ **Female**

Table No. 2
Distribution of young adults according to Mizaj
(n=100)

Mizaj	No. of adults	Percentage (%)
Damvi	13	13.00
Balghami	28	28.00
Safravi	53	53.00
Saudavi	06	6.00
Total	**100**	**100%**

Figure No. 2
Distribution of young adults according to Mizaj

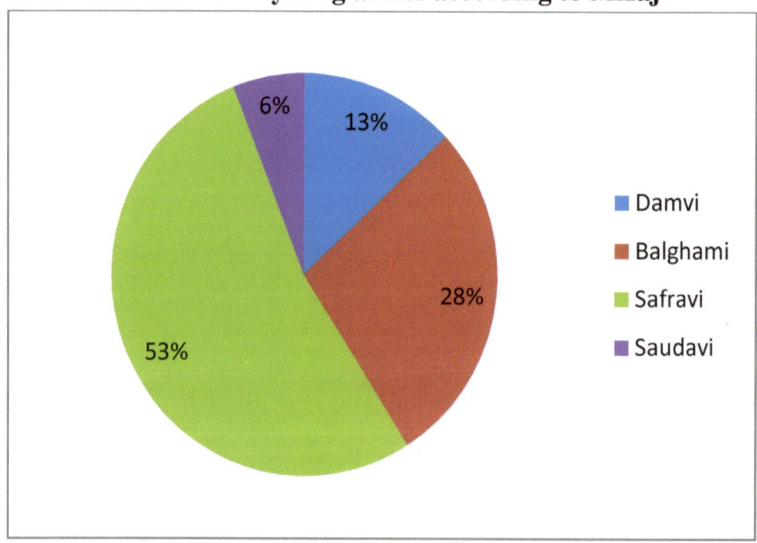

Table No. 3
Distribution of adults according to Religion
(n=100)

Religion	No. of Patients	Percentage (%)
Muslim	68	68.00
Hindu	30	30.00
Christian	2	2.00
Total	**100**	**100%**

Figure No. 3
Distribution of Adults according to Religion
(n=100)

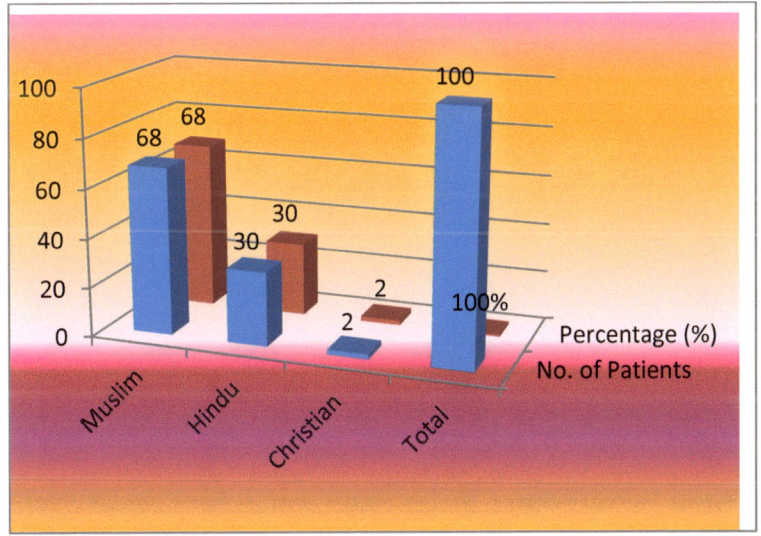

Table No. 4
Distribution of adults according to Habitual
(n=100)

Habitual	No. of adults	Percentage (%)
Urban	74	74.00
Rural	13	13.00
Semi-urban	13	13.00
Total	**100**	**100%**

Figure No. 4
Distribution of Adults according to Habitual
(n=100)

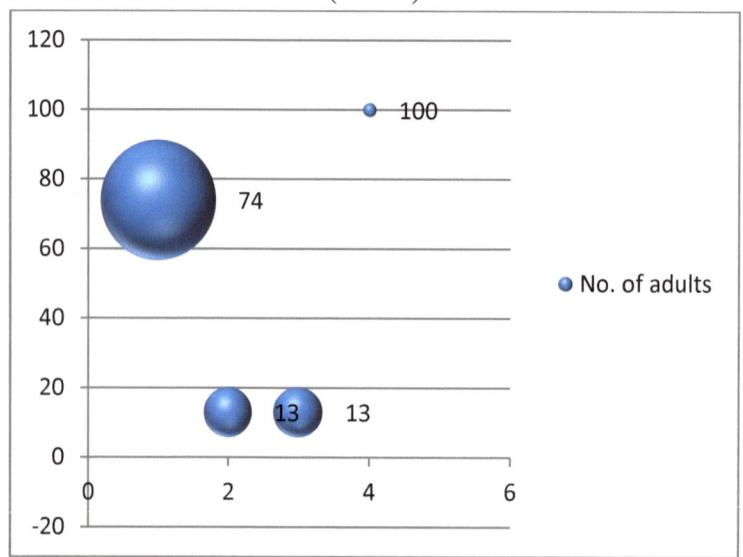

Table No. 5
Distribution of Patients according to Marital Status
(n=100)

Marital Status	No. of Adults	Percentage (%)
Married	14	14
Unmarried	86	86
Total	**100**	**100%**

Figure No. 5
Distribution of Adults according to Marital Status

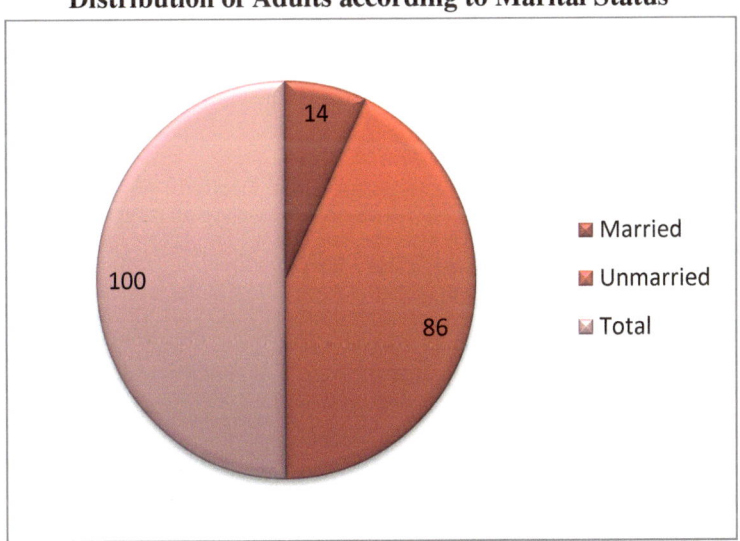

Table No. 6
Distribution of adults according to Family Type
(n=100)

Family	No. of adults	Percentage (%)
Nuclear	46	46.00
Joint	53	53.00
Broken	1	1.00
Total	**100**	**100%**

Figure No. 6
Distribution of Adults according to Family Type
(n=100)

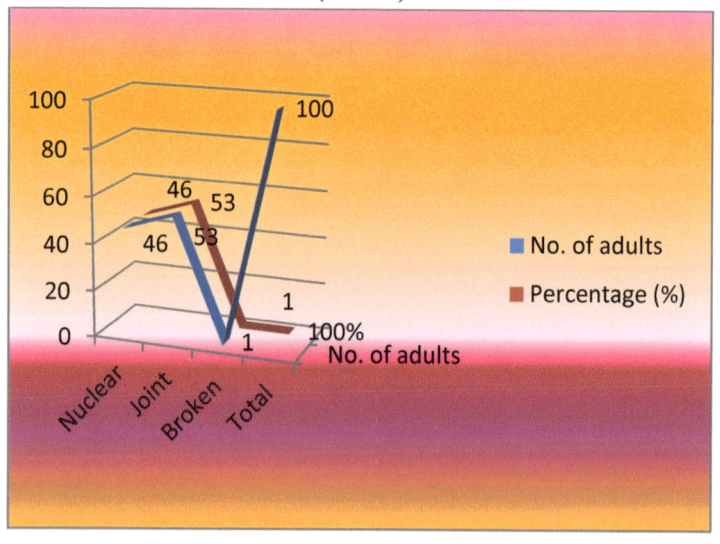

Table No. 7
Distribution of adults according to Diet Type
(n=100)

Diet	No. of adults	Percentage (%)
Vegetarian	18	18.00
Non-vegetarian	82	82.00
Total	**100**	**100%**

Figure No. 7
Distribution of Adults according to Diet Type
(n=100)

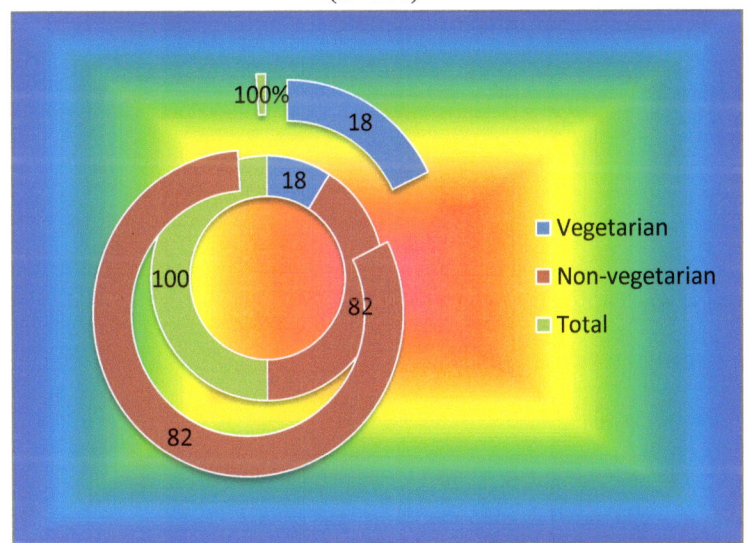

Table no 8

Distribution of Adults according to Socioeconomic Status (n=100)

Socioeconomic Status	No. of Patients	Percentage (%)
Upper	0	0.00
Upper middle	24	24.00
Lower middle	34	34.00
Upper lower	40	40.00
Lower	2	2.00
Total	**100**	**100%**

Figure No. 8

Distribution of Adults according to Socioeconomic Status

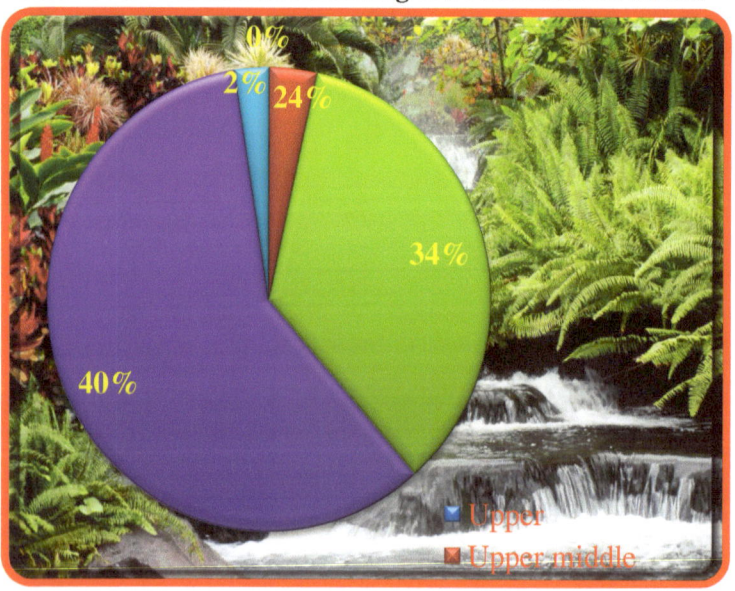

Table no 9
FVC Data summary assumption in different *Mizaj* adults

Group	Mean	Standard Deviation	Median
Mizaj Damvi	109.92	20.958	110.00
Balghami	109.79	20.495	102.00
Safravi	110.81	18.974	107.00
Saudavi	111.83	9.827	112.00

Figure no 9
FVC Data summary assumption in different *Mizaj* adults

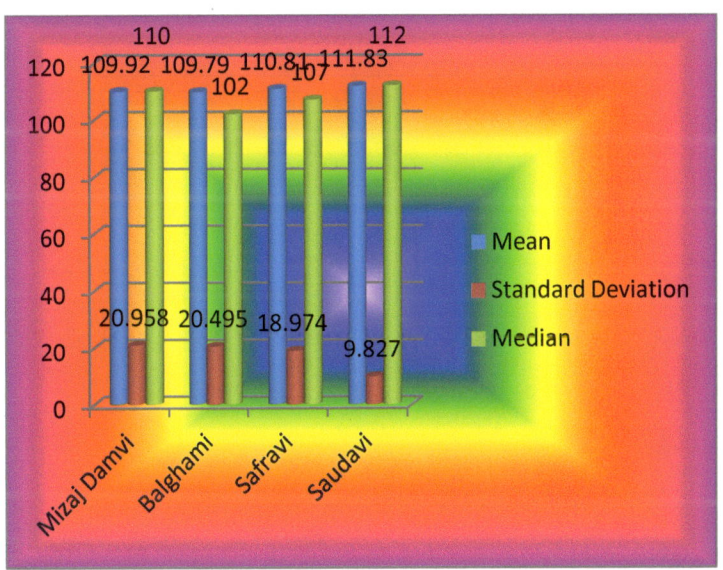

Table no 10

FEV1 Data summary assumption in different *Mizaj* adults

Group	Mean	Standard Deviation	Median
Mizaj Damvi	100.69	17.437	100.00
Balghami	109.79	20.495	102.00
Safravi	103.42	15.981	100.00
Saudavi	106.33	11.343	105.50

Figure no 10

FEV1 Data summary assumption in different *Mizaj* adults

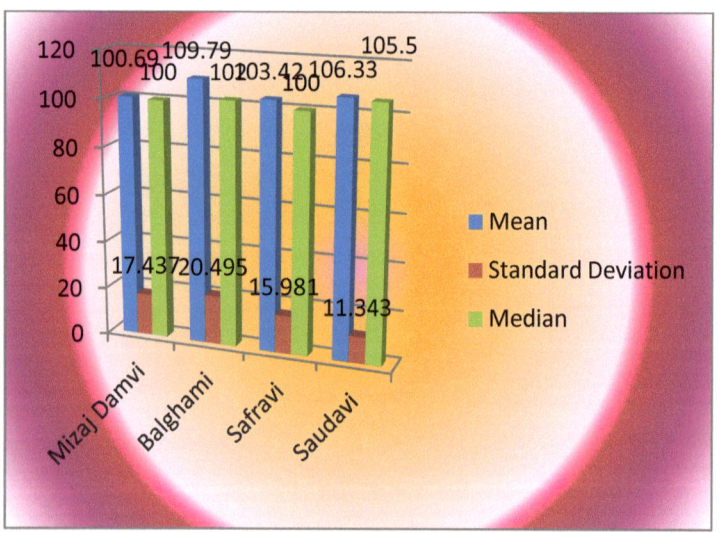

Table no 11

PEFR Data summary assumption in different _Mizaj_ adults

Group	Mean	Standard Deviation	Median
Mizaj Damvi	106.08	15.650	106.00
Balghami	107.54	27.296	103.50
Safravi	108.04	27.189	106.00
Saudavi	120.64	17.131	113.50

Figure no 11

PEFR Data summary assumption in different _Mizaj_ adults

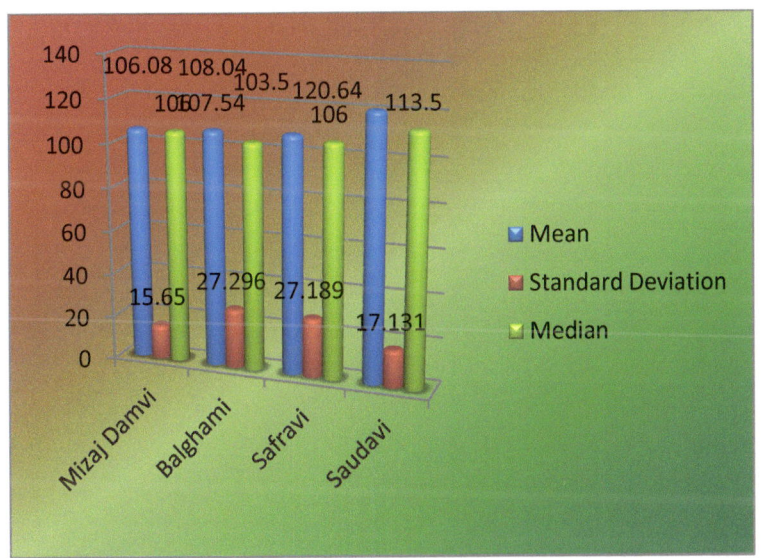

DISCUSSION

In the Unani system of medicine, *Mizaj* is one of the basic principles regarding diagnosis and making line of treatment of the disease. *Mizaj* is the *Kaifiyat* (quality) produced in the *Murakkab* (compound) by intermixing and interaction of *Ustaqissate Arba'* with their equal or unequal quantities. Human being is also considered as a *Murakkab* and gets its temperament in uterus in the form of *Nutfa* (zygote) after intermixing of *Maadda e Manviyah*. These *Maadda e Manviyah* are also made from *Ustaqissate Arba'* i.e. *Juze Nari, Maee, Hawaee* and *Juze Arzi*. The temperament furnished to the foetus makes it capable for the survival and development during foetal life as well as in the external environment (out of the uterus). If a child is furnished with *Mizaje Asli* as *Mo'tadil* he adjusts himself properly as per environmental demands and will survive and vice versa. It is clear from the definition of health that health is the manifestation of correctness of *Mizaj*. In other words, health is the name of proper functioning of the body that is impossible in the absence of *Mizaj e Mo'tadil* (good temperament). There are some factors responsible for changing the temperament of an individual i.e. age, weather, *Masakin* (residence), *Tadabeer,* occupation and habit of an individual. Like WHO, Unani system of medicine has also a goal for maintaining health of mankind and in this regard, it has been serving to the humanity for centuries.

To improve the health status of a country it is necessary to improve health of a community at individual level, which is impossible without knowing about *Halate Badan* (diseased and healthy condition of body) of an individual. The *Halaate Badan* are recognized by the temperament of an individual. Eminent Unani physicians have described two standards, which are used for this purpose. These scales or measurements are used to assess the temperament, by which we can make a diagnosis of disease and may be aware about condition of the body of an individual. This measurement is comprised of 10 *A'lamat* (determinants) known as *Ajnase A'shra*. Out of which some give information about the *Sakht* (structure) and others about the functions of the body. As *Mizaj* is measured on the basis of two criteria i.e. *Mizaj e Khilti* and *Mizaj e Khilqi* therefore, two proforma have been used to assess the temperament in present study, one was concerned with *Mizaje Khilqi*, and the other was for the determination of *Mizaj e Khilti* which is comprised of signs and symptoms of dominance of *Akhlate Badan*.

If these two standards or scales applied properly *Mizaj* of an individual may be determined accurately and then we may know about the *Haalat e Badan* (body conditions) and can predict about the diseases that may occur in the body in future and what type of precautions should be adopted for maintaining health.

Keeping these points in mind this study was conducted. Present cross-sectional study was carried out in Ayurvedic and Unani Tibbia College, Karol Bagh, New Delhi on 100 healthy individuals as per specially designed protocol which is mentioned in methodology. After enrolment of the individuals their temperament was assessed. Following assessment of *Mizaj* an attempt was made to correlate between *Mizaj* of individual and of the pulmonary functions. Findings/ observations regarding demographic data and *Mizaj* were as follows:

As shown in table no. 1, out of total individuals, 67% were male and 33% were female. The data revealed relatively higher number of individuals in male group then in female group. By these data temperamental correlation is not possible; simply the observed number may be because of higher number of male individuals in said group of the college. Out of total 100 individuals, 67 (67.00%) were males and 33 (33.00%) individuals were females. The difference may be due to easy access and high health consciousness in male as compared to female as females are less educated in India.

As shown in table no. 2, out of the total individuals of *Mizaj Damvi*, 13 were found in the study group, 28 were found *Mizaj Balghami, 53 were found Mizaj Safravi* and 6 were found *Mizaj* Saudavi. The data showed higher prevalence (53%) of individuals with *Mizaj Safravi in* the study group. Since the present study is first of its own type, so, the contemporary data were not available in this regard for comparison. *Sinne Shabab* is said as *Har Yabis* age, so in this age (18-30 years), prevalence and susceptibility to *Har Mizaj* of the individuals should be higher and so it is.

As shown in Table 3, In the present study, out of 100 individuals, Religion wise distribution of individuals revealed that out of the total 100 individuals in the study 30(30.00%) individuals were Hindu, 68(68.00%) were Muslim, and 2(2.00%) were Christian. The area of the study was Muslim dominated so Muslim preference was inevitable.

As shown in Table 4, out of 100 individuals, 74(74.00%) were urban, 13(13.00%) were rural, and 13(13.00%) were from semi urban. Higher prevalence of urban individuals was found in the study as compared to rural and semi urban individual prevalence.

As shown in Table 5, out of 100 individuals 86(86.00%) were unmarried, and 14(14.00%) were married. There was a higher prevalence of unmarried compare to married individuals.

As shown in Table 6, in the present study out of total 100 individuals 46(46.00%) individuals belonged to nuclear family, 53(53.00%) belonged to joint family and 1(1.00%) belonged to broken family. Maximum numbers of 53(53.00%) individuals belonged to joint family.

As shown in Table 7, in the present study out of total 100 individuals 18(18.00%) were vegetarian and 82(82.00%) were non-vegetarian. Maximum numbers of 82(82.00%) individuals were found non-vegetarian in the study.

As shown in Table 8, Out of total 100 individuals in the study 24(24.00 %) individuals were belonging to upper middle (2) SES, 34(34.00%%) individuals were belonging to lower middle (3) SES, and 40(40.00%) individuals were belonging to upper lower (4) SES. Maximum numbers, 40(40.00%) individuals were belonging to upper lower (4) SES.

In different Mizaj individuals, FVC assumption is done, P value found 0.9927, considered not significant. Variation among mean is not significantly greater than expected by chance. ANOVA assumes that the data is sampled from population with identical SDs. So this assumption is tested using the method of Bartlett (Table No.9).

Bartlett statistics corrected value is found 3.329, and P value 0.3436. This test suggests that the difference among SDs is not significant.

ANOVA assumes that the data are sampled from population that follow Gaussian distributions. This assumption is tested using the Kolmogorov and Smirnov as of follows:

Group	KS	P value	Passed normality test
Damvi	0.1718	>0.10	Yes
Balghami	0.2011	0.0052	No
Safravi	0.1296	0.0266	No
Saudavi	0.2005	>0.10	Yes

In different Mizaj individuals, FEV1 value assumpted, P value found 0.3386, considered not significant. Variation among mean is not significantly greater than expected by chance. ANOVA assumes that the data is sampled from population with identical SDs. So this assumption is tested using the method of Bartlett (Table No.10).

Bartlett statistics corrected value is found 3.601, and P

value 0.3079. This test suggests that the difference among SDs is not significant.

ANOVA assumes that the data are sampled from population that follow Gaussian distributions. This assumption is tested using the Kolmogorov and Smirnov as of follows:

Group	KS	P value	Passed normality test
Damvi	0.1429	>0.10	Yes
Balghami	0.2011	0.0052	No
Safravi	0.1397	0.0115	No
Saudavi	0.2687	>0.10	Yes

In different Mizaj individuals, for interpretation of PEFR value results one way of analysis (ANOVA) is applied, it assumes that the data are sampled from population with identical SDs. This assumption was tested by using the method of Bartlett.

Bartlett statistic corrected value was found 5.959 and P value is >0.05. Bartlett test suggests that the difference among the SDs is not significant (Table no.11).

ANOVA assumes that data are sampled from populations that follow Gaussian distributions. This assumption is tested using the method Kolmogorov and Smirnov.

Group	KS	P Value	Passed normality test
Damvi	0.1657	>0.10	Yes
Balghami	0.1783	0.0229	No
Safravi	0.1403	0.0109	No
Saudavi	0.2963	>0.10	Yes

In the present study, our emphasis was on *Mizaj* of the individual and *its relationship with pulmonary functions in various types of mizaj* were found normal in all types of Mizaj of healthy young individuals, therefore, the observed concordance between *Mizaj* and pulmonary functions distribution may be attributed to those factors which tend to alter the *Mizaj* and have potential to produce diseases like, *Mizaj e Khilqi*, age, *Masakin* (residence), weather, diets, occupation and habit.

Further study on a large scale is needed to determine relationship and concordance between *Mizaj* and pulmonary functions considering these factors along with *Mizaj*.

CONCLUSION

Out of total individuals, 67% were male and 33% were female. The data revealed relatively higher number of individuals in male group whereas lower number in female group. By these data temperamental correlation is not possible; simply the observed number may be because of higher number of male individuals in said group of the college. Out of total 100 individuals, 67 (67.00%) were males and 33 (33.00%) individuals were females. The difference may be due to easy access and high health consciousness in male as compared to female.

Out of the total individuals, 13 were found of *Mizaj Damvi* in the study group, 28 were found *Mizaj Balghami, 53 were found Mizaj Safravi* and 6 were found *Mizaj Saudavi*. The data showed higher prevalence (53%) of individuals with *Mizaj Safravi i*n the study group.

In the present study, out of 100 individuals, religion wise distribution of individuals revealed that out of the total 100 individuals in the study 30(30.00%) individuals were Hindu, 68(68.00%) were Muslim, and 2(2.00%) were Christian.

Out of 100 individuals, 74(74.00%) were urban, 13(13.00%) were rural, and 13(13.00%) were from semi urban. Higher prevalence of urban individuals was found in the study as compared to rural and semi urban individual prevalence.

Out of 100 individuals 86(86.00%) were unmarried, and 14(14.00%) were married. A higher prevalence of unmarried compare to married individuals.

In the present study out of total 100 individuals 46(46.00%) individuals were belonging to nuclear family, 53(53.00%) were belonging to joint family and 1(1.00%) were belonging to broken family. Maximum numbers of 53(53.00%) individuals were belonging to joint family.

In the present study out of total 100 individuals

76

18(18.00%) were vegetarian and 82(82.00%) were non-vegetarian. Maximum numbers of 82(82.00%) individuals were found non-vegetarian in the study.

Out of total 100 individuals in the study 24(24.00 %) individuals were belonging to upper middle (2) SES, 34(34.00%) individuals were belonging to lower middle (3) SES, and 40(40.00%) individuals were belonging to upper lower (4) SES. Maximum numbers, 40(40.00%) individuals were belonging to upper lower (4) SES.

In different Mizaj individuals, FVC assumption is done, P value found 0.9927, considered not significant. Variation among mean is not significantly greater than expected by chance. ANOVA assumes that the data is sampled from population with identical SDs. So this assumption is tested using the method of Bartlett.

Bartlett statistics corrected value is found 3.329, and P value 0.3436. This test suggests that the difference among SDs is not significant.

In different *Mizaj* individuals, FEV1 value assumpted, P value found 0.3386, considered not significant. Variation among mean is not significantly greater than expected by chance. ANOVA assumes that the data is sampled from population with identical SDs. So this assumption is tested using the method of Bartlett. Bartlett statistics corrected value is found 3.601, and P value 0.3079. This test suggests that the difference among SDs is not significant. ANOVA assumes that the data are sampled from population that follow Gaussian distributions.

In different Mizaj individuals, for interpretation of PEFR value results one way of analysis (ANOVA) is applied, it assumes that the data are sampled from population with identical SDs. This assumption was tested by using the method of Bartlett. Bartlett statistic corrected value was found 5.959 and P value is >0.05. Bartlett test suggests that the difference among the SDs is not significant.

REFERENCES:

1. Pierce, R. (2005). "Spirometry: An essential clinical measurement". Australian family physician 34 (7): 535–539
2. Renzetti AD Jr. Standardization of spirometry. Am Rev Respir Dis 1979; 119: 831–838.
3. American Academy of Allergy, Asthma, and Immunology, "Five Things Physicians and Patients Should Question", Choosing Wisely: an initiative of the ABIM Foundation (American Academy of Allergy, Asthma, and Immunology), retrieved 14 August 2013
4. Surgeryencyclopedia.com, Spirometry tests. Retrieved 14 Sept 2013
5. Stanojevic S, Wade A, Stocks J, et al. (February 2008). Reference Ranges for Spirometry Across All Ages: A New Approach. Am. J. Respir. Crit. Care Med. 177 (3): 253–60
6. Perez, LL (March–April 2013). "Office spirometry". Osteopathic Family Physician 5 (2): 65–69
7. Lung function, Practice compendium for semester (VI). Department of Medical Sciences, Clinical Physiology, Academic Hospital, Uppsala, Sweden
8. Hedenström H. Interpretation model compendium at Uppsala Academic Hospital: 2009
9. Nunn AJ, Gregg I (April 1989). New regression equations for predicting peak expiratory flow in adults. BMJ 298 (6680): 1068–70.
10. George, Ronald B. (2005). Chest medicine: essentials of pulmonary and critical care medicine. Lippincott Williams & Wilkins. p. 96
11. Townsend, MC. American College of occupational and Environmental Medicine (ACOEM) Position Statement: Evaluating Pulmonary Function Change Over Time in the Occupational Setting. JOEM; 47:1307-1316, 2005.
12. Third National Health and Nutrition Examination Survey III:SpirometryProcedure Manual.http://www.cdc.gov/nchs/about/major/nhanes/NHANESIII_Reference_Manuals.

13. Hankinson, J.L., Odencrantz, J.R., and Fedan, K.B. (1999). Spirometric reference values from a sample of the general U.S. population. Am J Respir Crit Care Med, 159, 179-187.

14. Tabri R. *Firdausul Hikmat* (Urdu Translation). Deoband: Faisal Publication; 2002: 52, 6,101,107,122,128.

15. Majoosi A. *Kamilus Sana'ah* (Urdu Translation by Kantoori GH). Vol. 1. Lucknow: Munshi Nawal Kishore; 1889: 25-28.

16. Kabeeruddin M. *Kulliyate Qanoon* (Urdu Translation) Vol.1. New Delhi: Aijaz Publishing House; 2007: 20-56.

17. Ibn Rushd AWM. *Kitabul Kulliyat* (Urdu translation by CCRUM). 2nd ed. New Delhi: CCRUM; 1987: 146-157,356-361,358.

18. Chandpuri K. *Moojazal Qanoon*. 3rd ed. New Delhi: Qaumi Council Barae Farogh Urdu Zaban; 1998: 45-47.

19. Ibn Sina. *Alqanoon fit Tib* (Urdu Translation by Kantoori GH). Vol.1. New Delhi: Idara Kitabul Shifa; 2007: 17.

20. Narain, "Health care of Temperaments & constitutional Defects" , 2nd Edition, Shri Satguru Publishers , Delhi, 1996, pp. xi ,xii.

21. Jalinoos. *Kitabu fil Firaqi Tib* (Urdu Translation by Zillur Rehman). Aligarh: Ibn Sina Academy; 2000: 75-76.

22. Azmi, A.A., " Basic concept of Unani Medicine- Acritical study", 1st Edition, Jamia Hamdard, New Delhi, 1995, pp. 57,58 , 59 ,61 ,62, 73, 77, 78, 98, 99, 106.

23. Glynn, John p. , "Temperaments Revisited- New Interest in an old concept" at www.e-imj.com/Vol2-No2/vol2-No2-N2.htm

24. Majusi,Ali Ibn Abbas, "Kamil-us-Sana-part 1", Urdu translation by Ghulam Hussain kantoori, Matab Munshi Naval Kishore, Lucknow, 1989, pp. ,24 ,25 ,42.

25. Masihi , Abu Sahel Isa Bin YAHya Bin Ibrahim, "Kitab -AL –Me'yah Fil Tibb- part -1, Islamic Publication Society Hyderabad (Deccan), 1963, p.82.

26. Zaidi, I.H. & Zulkifle, M. "Temperamentology : A Scientific Appraisal Of Human Temperaments" , 1st edition, Aligarh, 1999, pp.12,13,14,20,22,64.

27. Ibn-e-sina, Abu Ali hussain Bin Abdullah, "Al-Qanun Fil-Tibb Part-1," Urdu Translation by Ghulam Hussain Kantoori, Lucknow, 1303 Hijri, pp13, 152-157.

28. Jurjani , Ahmad –ul-Hasan, "Zakhira Khwazam Shahi vol. 1". Urdu translation by Hadi Hussain Khan, Matab Munshi Naval Kishore, Lucknow ,1902 p.16.

29. Ibn –e- Hubal, Abul Hasan Ali bin ahmad baghdadi, kitab-ul-Muktarat Fil- Tibb , part 1 Urdu translation bu CCRUM New Delhi 2005, p.23.

30. Ibn-e-Nafees, Burhanuddin Kirmani Ibn-e- Ooz, "Kulliyat-e-Nafisi Vol. 2," Urdu Translation & Elaboration (Shsrah) by Hakim M. Kabiruddin, Matba Daftar-Al- Maseeh, Bazar Noor-ul-Umra, hyderabad Deccan,1952, p. 19.

31. Antaqi, Daood , Bin Umar, " Tazkerat-ul-Albab vol. 1 matab ata al Zaharze Egypt, 1349 hijri, p.9 .

32. Khan , Mohd Iliyas, " Qanun Asri vol.1, Jayyad Barqi , Prees, Delhi, 1931, pp.41-47.

33. Gruner O.C " A Treatise on the canon of medicine of Avicenna", Luzac & company, London, pp.57,63,64, 242,246-273.

34. Falsafi , Abdul Latif, Shifa-ul-mulk "Tajdeed-e- Tibb", Matba Hakim Syed Zillur Rehman, Ala Press, Delhi, 1972, p.49.

35. Iqsarai, Mohd. Jamaluddin , Hal- al- Moajiz vol.1 Urdu translation by mohd Ayub Israili, Mataba Munshi Naval Kishore, Lucknow, 1907 p.3

36. Gazrooni, Sadeeduddin, "Kulliyat-e-sadidi," Translation by maulvi syed Abid Hussain, , Mataba Munshi Naval Kishore, Lucknow, 1911, pp.12, 13.

37. Latif, A., "A Temperament. In :Philosphy of medicine & Science," Compiled by Department of Philosphy of medicine & Science, IHMMR, New Delhi, 1972, p. 129.

38. Shah M.H " Temperaments: Explanations & Interpretations, In : Department of Philosphy of medicine & Science, IHMMR, New Delhi, 1972, p. 123-124.

39. Mehdi Hasan, S. " A rational Interpretation of the four cosmic elements as operating in Alchemy. In: theories & Philosophies of Medicine " 2nd edition IHMMR , New Delhi 1973 p.209.

40. Ahmad, S. Ishtiaq , " Introduction to Al-Umur Al-tabiyah ", 1st edition , Saini printers , New Delhi , 1980, pp.16, 17, 18 ,32, 37, 49, 50, 54, 55-58.

41. Taiyab, M., "Philosophy of Greeco-arabiain Medicine", A.M.U press, Aligarh. 1983 p.24.

42. Kirmani NBA. *Kulliate Nafeesi* (Urdu translation by Kabeeruddin M). Vol.1. New Delhi: Idara Kitabul Shifa; YNM: 19-80.

43. Ghulam J. *Makhzanul Jawahar*. New Delhi: Aijaz Publishing House; 1998: 797-800.

44. Ibnul Quf. *Kitabul U'mdah fil Jarahat* (Urdu translation by CCRUM). Lucknow. (Unit Lucknow); YNM: 18-30.

45. Rauf KAH, Anjum R. *Mizaj Advia Ki Scientific Tuazeeh. Jahane Tib* 2008; 9 (3): 35.

46. Brunwald E, Fauci AS, Kasper DL, Hauser SL, Longo DL, Jameson JL. Harrison's Principles of Internal Medicine. Vol.1. 15th ed. New Delhi: McGraw Hill; 2001: 1152-153.

47. Brunwald E, Fauci AS, Kasper DL, Hauser SL, Longo DL, Jameson JL. Harrison's Principles of Internal Medicine. Vol. 2. 15th ed. New Delhi: Mc Graw Hill; 2001: 1301

48. Hunter AAJ, Colledge RN, Boon AN, Chilvers RE, Christopher H. Davidson's Principle and Practice of Medicine. 19th ed. New Delhi: Churchill Livingstone; 2004: 340-42.

49. Park K. Park's Textbook of Preventive and Social Medicine. 19th ed. Jabalpur: M/S Banarsidas Bhanot; 2007: 462-466, 674-80.

50. Harsh M. Textbook of Pathology. 5th ed. New Delhi: Jaypee Brothers; 2005: 265.

51. Thomas CL. Taber's Cyclopedic Medical Dictionary. Vol.1. 18th ed. New Delhi: Jaypee Brothers; 1989: 571.

52. Thomas CL. Taber's Cyclopedic Medical Dictionary. Vol. 2. 18th ed. New Delhi: Jaypee Brothers; 1989:1464.

53. Timmreck TC. An Introduction to Epidemiology. 2nd ed. Massachusetts: Jones and Bartlett Publishers; 1998: 72-73.

54. Jurjani SI. *Zakhira Khwarzm Shahi* (Urdu Translation by Khan HH). Vol. 1. Lucknow: Munshi Nawal Kishore; 1996: 14-26.

55. Ibn Sina. *Al Qanoon fit Tib* (Urdu Translation by Kantoori GH). Vol. 4. New Delhi: Idara Kitabus Shifa; 2007: 1138.

56. Zaidi IH, Zulkifle M, Ahmad SN. Temperamentology- A scientific appraisal of human temperament. 1st ed. Aligarh: AMU; 1999: 22-23.

57. Ahmed SI. Introduction to *AL U*mur *al Tabiah*. 1st ed. New Delhi: Saini Printers; 1980: 140.

58. Amin MMW, Khan KZ, Ahmed S. *Mizaje Damvi ka Mutalea Imtehane Damvi ki Roshni Main*. Jahane Tib 2005; 6 (3): 29.

59. Majoosi A. *Kamilus Sana'ah* (Urdu Translation by Kintoori GH). Vol. 2. Lucknow: Munshi Nawal Kishore; 1889: 3-78.

PRO-FORMA FOR ASSESSMENT OF MIZAJ BY AJNAS E ASHRA
DEMOGRAPHIC PROFILE

Name of the Individual......................

Age/Sex............   Marital Status................

Religion / caste .... Education

...................Occupation ....

Income................   Contact

no......................................

Address

Parameter	Signs and Symptoms of			
	Mizaje Har	Mizaje Barid	Mizaje Ratab	Mizaje Yabis
1. Malmas (touch) Thermometer reading	hot	cold	soft and moist	hard and rough
	°F			
2. Mahm wa shahm (muscularity and adiposity)	Mid arm circumpherence cm			
	Skin fold thickness cm			
	good muscular development and less fat	deficient in musculature and excess in fat	good muscular and excess in fat	leanness (less muscles and less fat)
3. Badan ke Bal (hair) .growth .thickness .density .shape .color	rapid thick dense curly blackish	slow thin sparse straight brownish (onion) or absolutely red or	slow thin sparse straight whitish	Rapid Thick Dense curly whitish (grayish)

83

		redness tilt to yellow or white		
.no. of hair per 1 inch square area of skin on manubrium				
4.Badan ka rang (colour of body / complexion)	reddish-white (rosy)/ or color of wheat	whitish/purple	whitish (chalky	purple / blackish as color of lead
5. A'za ki Hayyat (physique) . skeleton	Broad chest , large and well developed hands and feet	Narrow chest, small And under developed hands and feet	Broad chest , large and well developed hands and feet	Narrow chest, small And under developed hands and feet
. veins on body	Prominent and of wide caliber	Not prominent , not of wide caliber, soft	Prominent, narrow and soft	Narrow and hard
. pulse and breath	strong and large volume pulse and deep breath	weak and small volume pulse and slow breath	strong and large volume pulse and fast deep breath	Small pulse and Slow breath
.muscles around the joints	good muscular	less	good	less muscular developme

84

	development, specially around the joints	muscular development	muscular development, specially around the joints	nt
.body joints .facial features	most prominent sharp – lips, nose etc	buried	most buried	prominent sharp – lips, nose etc
6. A'za ka jald ya bader mutassir hona . well toleration for .comparatively remain well in	cold winter	heat summer	dryness autumn	dampness rainy season
7. Neend wa Bedari (sleep and wake fullness) . sleep habit (when you want to sleep) . wakefulness .sleep duration	Get it hardly Get it easily normal sleep duration	get it easily get it hardly Sound sleep duration	get it easily get it hardly increased sleep duration	get it hardly get it hardly decreased sleep duration
	sleep duration		Hours	

8. Af'ale A'za (functiona state of organ)				
. body movement	active	dull	hypoactive	hyper active
	fast and continuous	slow		
. talking	strong and loud	weak and high pitch		
. speech				
. blinking of eyes per minute	rapid	Slow	Moderate	Slow
. growth of organ, hair	reddish	Whitish	Whitish	Greyish
. colour of eyes	oily and salty (cold , dry)	Sweet (hot and dry)	Vegetarian (cold and mixed)	Non-vegetarian (hot and moist)
. diet (most liked)	above normal (good)	normal	Sub normal	Hyper
. appetite				
9. Fuzlate Badan	reddish with strong smell concentrated	white or colourless and decreased smell	white or colourless and decreased smell	Dark and concentrated
. urine				
. stool				hard with decreased smell
	soft with strong smell strong odour	soft with decreased smell weak odour	soft with decreased smell	
. sweet				
10. Infia'alate Nafsaniah (psychologic				

al activity)

	Aggressive	non-aggressive	Less aggressive	Hardly aggressive
1.To external stimuli and adverse condition	Aggressive	non-aggressive	Less aggressive	Hardly aggressive
2. power of mental conception	easily conceive	hardly conceive	Not easily conceive	Very hardly conceive
3.memory	short term memory	long term memory	short term memory	long term memory
4.thinking	bright and hopeful	afraid of being something wrong	less bright and hopeful	very afraid of being something wrong
5.anger	more	less	for short period	for long period
6.bravery	more	less	for short period	for long period
7.intelligence	more	less	not more	for long period
8.hopefull	more	less	not more	very less
9.fear	absent	less	not more	very less
		more	for short period	very less
				persistent

Signature of PG Scholar

SIGNS AND SYMPTOMS OF DOMINANCE OF AKHLAT DAM (BLOOD)

1 .Feelings of Heaviness in the Body, Specially, Behind the Eyes and over

the Head and Temporal Region (Temples)
[YES/NO]

2. Stretching and /or Yawing are Frequent
[YES/NO]

3. Excessive Tendency to Drowsiness and Sleep Perception is Poor [YES/NO]

4. Fatigue is Felt Even without Exertion
[Yes/No]

5. Sweet Taste in the Mouth Often Without Cause
[Yes/No]

6. Tongue Is Usually Red
[Yes/No]

7. Boils on the Body and Ulcers on Tongue Are Common
[Yes/No]

8. Bleeding From the Gums Nostrils and Anus
[Yes/No]

9. Red Things Flowing Of Blood, Immersed / Sung In Blood in Dream [Yes/No]

BALGHAM (PHLEGM)

1. Excessive pallor, flabbiness of body
   [yes/no]

2. Cold and moist skin
   [yes/no]

3. Excessive salivation and viscid saliva
   [yes/no]

4. Diminished thirst, except when the acid phlegm
   [yes/no]

5. Weak digestion with acid eructation
   [yes/no]

6. Pale urine
   [yes/no]

7. Excessive sleepiness
   [yes/no]

8. Flabby muscles
   [yes/no]

9. Mental dullness
   [yes/no]

10. Soft pulse of slow rate and speed
    [yes/no]

11. Dream about water, canals cold ice and thundering hail-
storms   [yes/no]

SAFRA (BILE)

1. yellow colour of eyes and complexion
   [yes/no]
2. rough and dry tongue, nostrils
   [yes/no]
3. desire for cold breezes
   [yes/no]
4. excessive thirst
   [yes/no]
5. lack of appetite
   [yes/no]
6. nausea with bilious vomiting of green or yellow colour
   [yes/no]
7. bitter taste in mouth
   [yes/no]
8. irritative diarrhoea
   [yes/no]
9. seeing fire in dream
   [yes/no]
10. seeing of flags of yellow colour
    [yes/no]
11. rapid pulse
    [yes/no]
12. things looking yellow (which are not yellow)
    [yes/no]
13. feeling of burning and irritation in the body as from hot bath

    or exposure to the sun
    [yes/no]

SAUDA (BLACK BILE)

1. dry and dark skin
         [yes /no]
2. anxiety
      [yes/no]
3. burning in the epigestrium
         [yes/no]
4. false appetite
      [yes/no]
5. thick and turbid urine of blue, black or red colour
         [yes/no]
6. dark complexion
      [yes/no]
7. excessive hairiness
      [yes/no]
8. excess of thinking
      [yes/no]
9. waswas
      [yes/no]
10. dreams usually full of anxiety as dark places, dark trenches
    and dark fearful objects
         [yes/no]

Signature of PG Scholar

Kuppuswamy's Socioeconomic Status Scale

Score Card	
A. Education	**Score**
1 Professional	7
2 Graduate or post graduate	6
3 Intermediate or post high school diploma	5
4 High school certificate	4
5 Middle school certificate	3
6 Primary school certificate	2
7 Illiterate	1
B. Occupation	**Score**
1 Professional	10
2 Semi professional	6
3 Clerical, shop owner, farmer	5
4 Skilled worker	4
5 Semiskilled worker	3
6 Unskilled worker	2
7 Unemployed	1
C. Family income per month (in Rs.)	**Score**
1 $\geq$19575	12
2 9788-19574	10
3 7323-9787	6
4 4894-7322	4
5 2936-4893	3
6 980-2935	2
7 $\leq$979	1
Total Scores	**Socioeconomic status**
26-29	Upper (I)

16-25	Upper Middle (II)
11-15	Lower Middle (III)
5-10	Upper Lower (IV)
≤ 5	Lower (V)

Authored: Dr Danish Kamal Chishti
Designed by: Dr Izharul Hasan
Supervisor: Prof Yusuf Jamal
Co-supervisor: Dr Shabbir Ahmad
ISBN-10: 150598758X
ISBN-13: 978-1505987584
Product Dimensions: 6 x 9 inches
Pages: 94
Print: IS Independent, CA, Made in USA

www.ingramcontent.com/pod-product-compliance
Lightning Source LLC
Chambersburg PA
CBHW040827180526
45159CB00001B/97